Fit from the Start

How to Prevent Childhood Obesity in Infancy

Alvin N. Eden, MD

Barbara J. Moore, PhD

Adrienne Forman, MS, RDN

Fit from the Start: How to Prevent Childhood Obesity in Infancy
Alvin N. Eden, Barbara J. Moore, and Adrienne Forman

Published by Shape Up America!®

Paperback Edition:	978-0-9915302-2-9
EPUB Edition:	978-0-9915302-1-2
Kindle Edition:	978-0-9915302-0-5

Shape Up America!®
PO Box 149
Clyde Park, MT 59018
www.shapeup.org

Shape Up America!® and the authors are providing the information in this book solely as an educational resource. Shape Up America!® and the authors do not warrant or guarantee, and hereby disclaim, the accuracy, completeness, or timeliness of any information contained in the book. In no event shall Shape Up America!® and the authors be liable for any information included in or omitted from this book, or for any decision made or action taken by you in reliance on such information.

The information contained in this book does not constitute and should not be considered medical advice. For questions about your health or the health of a family member, you should consult an appropriately licensed clinician who can apply his or her professional judgment to the specific clinical circumstances presented by you or your family member.

The Shape Up America!® name and Shape Up America!® logo are registered trademarks of Shape Up America!®, a 501(c)3 nonprofit organization.

This book is dedicated to the memory of
C. Everett Koop, MD, ScD, the 13th Surgeon General of the
United States and the founder of Shape Up America!®

fit

from the

start

How to Prevent Childhood Obesity in Infancy

Alvin N. Eden, **MD** · Barbara J. Moore, **PhD**
Adrienne Forman, **MS, RDN**

Contents

Foreword

As I read this book, it struck me that had my husband, C. Everett Koop, lived just one more year, he would have so enjoyed reading it. I have no doubt he would have been very proud of this book and so pleased to have it dedicated to his memory.

Young people reading this book may not be aware how Dr. Koop established his professional reputation in the 1950s in the new field of pediatric surgery. Parents brought their newborn children with birth defects to him, hoping he might be able to fix the problems. Many of the defects were so unusual they did not even have names. Often, the operations he performed had never been attempted.

Dr. Koop and his team figured out how to anesthetize these tiny babies. Using pioneering techniques, they operated on 1,200 babies over the first several years and never lost one. But they sometimes had to sit up all night with their patients to coax them through recovery.

Toward the end of his tenure as U.S. Surgeon General (1981–1989), Dr. Koop became aware of the rapidly growing prevalence of obesity in America. The alarming data spurred him to found Shape Up America!® in 1994 to raise awareness of obesity as an important health issue.

As a surgeon who dedicated himself to relieving the suffering of children, he was greatly concerned about the 12 million children in America who are obese and the 2.5 million children who are severely obese. If he were alive today, I know he would join me in calling upon all parents and parents-to-be to read this book and learn how they can play a vital role in preventing childhood obesity.

Cora Hogue Koop
Hanover, New Hampshire
June 2014

Meet the Authors

Alvin Eden, MD, FAAP*

As a practicing pediatrician for over 40 years, I've seen increasing numbers of overweight and obese children. In 1975 I published my first book to address the problem, *Growing Up Thin*. The main theme was the treatment of the obese child. The book was a commercial success, but the prevalence of childhood obesity continued to increase, along with all the adverse health consequences, including more and more children developing type 2 diabetes.

After *Growing Up Thin* was published, I appeared on many national TV shows as an "expert" in treating obese children. Besides caring for the kids in my office, I was asked to treat large numbers of obese children sent to me by other physicians. As clinical professor of pediatrics at Weill Cornell Medical College in New York City, I have had the opportunity to share these experiences with many of my colleagues, pediatric residents and students.

But treatment isn't the answer; prevention is. New scientific data show the critical importance of preventing obesity during the very early years. If your child is obese when he enters kindergarten, chances are high that he will remain so.

Given current trends, it has become increasingly clear that to stem the childhood obesity epidemic we need to prevent it from happening in the first place. That's why we wrote *Fit from the Start: How to Prevent Childhood Obesity in Infancy*. Prevention starts before pregnancy and continues through pregnancy, infancy, toddlerhood and the preschool years. This book covers infancy—the first 12 months of life.

We hope this information will help you raise a healthy weight, active and happy baby who, in a few years, will enter school ready to learn, make friends and have fun.

* Fellow of the American Academy of Pediatrics

Barbara J. Moore, PhD, FTOS*

My professional career as an obesity research scientist began 35 years ago when I carried out my first study of childhood obesity while a graduate student at Columbia University. For nearly two decades I have served as the president and CEO of a nonprofit organization, Shape Up America!®, founded by a famous pediatric surgeon, C. Everett Koop, MD, ScD. Dr. Koop was appointed 13th U.S. Surgeon General by President Ronald Reagan (1981–1989), and for years after he left that office, people still regarded him as the "nation's doctor." Dr. Koop passed away in February 2013. But he enthusiastically supported the work required to develop a series of books intended to prevent childhood obesity.

It's in honor of Dr. Koop and his dedication to fostering good health in all people, especially children, that I embarked on this project. It is a labor of love.

Parents have the most important job in the world—raising healthy, well-adjusted kids. There are many factors that can undermine efforts to keep kids at a healthy weight as they grow. These include lack of health insurance for millions of American children, marketing messages that encourage children to consume unhealthful foods and beverages, and screen-based games that draw them away from outdoor, active play. Despite these challenges, there are things you can do while your child is still an infant to help keep obesity at bay.

This book concentrates on the factors that are within your control during this critical period of your child's life. You can help shape your baby's brain and behavioral development to minimize the risk of your child becoming obese later in life. Within the limits of current science and the constraints of today's society, this book will show you how.

* *Fellow of The Obesity Society*

Adrienne Forman, MS, RDN*

I have been a registered dietitian nutritionist working in weight management and nutrition communications for 25 years. My involvement with Shape Up America!® spans 15 years and I'm currently the director of nutrition communications. As a senior nutritionist with Weight Watchers in the 1990s, and a child weight-management specialist for over five years with MEND (Mind, Exercise, Nutrition…Do it!), the world's largest community-based child weight-management program, I've seen firsthand how adults and children can change their lifestyles and behaviors to successfully control their weight and improve their self-esteem.

Yet, wouldn't it be better if children didn't have to deal with the challenges of being overweight or obese in the first place? Wouldn't it be wonderful if parents could help their children, as young as infants, be healthy, active and happy, as well as free from obesity-related illness as they grow older? That's where prevention steps in. And that's the key reason we wrote *Fit from the Start: How to Prevent Childhood Obesity in Infancy.*

The foods that you and your baby eat affect how the appetite centers in your baby's brain develop and shape your child's taste preferences. By tuning in to your baby's hunger and satiety cues, you can avoid overfeeding. This will help your growing child stay at a healthy weight.

We want your baby to get a healthy start in life. We hope this book will help you make that happen.

* *Registered dietitian nutritionist, also called registered dietitian (RD)*

Acknowledgments

We would like to thank our colleagues at Shape Up America!® for their valuable insights and assistance in the development of this book: Joanna Barajas, Alex Colcord and Pat Fuchs. We are also grateful to Stephanie Cook for her helpful suggestions and to Alexa Greist, Heather Kern, Zulaikha Losman, Rachel Quenzer, Daria Segalini, Danielle Stember and Shana Wilkenfeld for taking the time to offer their new-mom perspectives on the content in this book.

Many thanks to Patricia Leffingwell for her illustrations and to Kristin Hammargren for creating, managing and playing a lead role in the infant exercise videos. We appreciate the skills of the videographer, Mike Kvackay. We also extend a big thanks to the moms, dad and adorable babies who co-starred in the videos: Jennifer Handy and her baby, Penelope; Frannie Moulton and her baby, Mary Pierce; Catherine Savery and her baby, Adam; Timothy Schober and his baby, Amelia.

We appreciate the guidance and publishing expertise of Saul Bottcher and Nas Hedron of IndieBookLauncher.com and the promotional skills of Dee Donavanik and Sandy Trupp of Media Connect. We are grateful for their time, talent and assistance in helping us publish and promote our book. Many thanks!

A Few Notes

This book focuses on what you can do to prevent your baby from becoming overweight or obese later in life. It's not intended to be a book about how to feed or care for your baby. There are excellent books available that address these topics in detail, and we recommend some in the Resources section at the end of this book.

The information in this book isn't a substitute for the care and advice of your baby's pediatrician or other healthcare provider. Regular check-ups are very important to protect the health and well-being of your child. We encourage you to discuss the information in this book, especially "Rapid Weight Gain—A Risk Factor for Childhood Obesity" on page 65, with your child's healthcare provider.

The information presented in this book applies equally to boys and girls, unless stated otherwise. To make the text easier to read, the chapters alternate between feminine and masculine pronouns.

We realize there are many types of caregivers. *Any reference to parents also applies to partners, grandparents, day care providers, nannies and any others who are responsible for the routine care and feeding of your baby.*

Introduction

Congratulations on the new addition to your family! Along with the joy you're experiencing, you may be feeling overwhelmed by the changes and responsibilities that parenthood brings. Chances are you're eager to do whatever it takes to help your baby grow up healthy and strong. That should include doing what you can to prevent your baby from reaching a weight that puts her future health at risk.

It's true that a certain amount of fat on a baby is normal and healthy. But having too much fat can lead to health and weight problems later on. Obesity among toddlers has more than doubled in the past 30 years. For some of these children, their excess fat was evident at birth; for others, it developed during infancy—the first 12 months of life. Although some obese infants will outgrow their obesity, a higher proportion will remain at an unhealthy weight.

There are things you can do now to help keep your baby from gaining too much weight too fast. What you eat, how you feed your baby, and how much sleep your baby gets can make a difference in her future weight.

The Time to Act is Now

In early 2014, the *New England Journal of Medicine* published a headline-making study showing that the first few years of a child's life are a critical time for preventing obesity. The researchers found that the likelihood of childhood obesity takes hold by the time children are 5 years old. Further, overweight kindergartners were four times more likely to be obese in eighth grade than children who weren't overweight when starting school.

This important study involved nearly 7,800 children, a sample that represented all the children in the United States who began kindergarten in 1998.

Researchers measured the children's height and weight seven times between kindergarten and eighth grade.

The results were startling. By the time the children entered kindergarten, over 12 percent were already obese; another 15 percent were overweight. Nearly 2 out of 3 obese children entering kindergarten remained obese through eighth grade and almost half of the overweight 5-year-olds became obese by age 14.

Many efforts to curb childhood obesity target school-aged children. But this study shows that, for many children, it may be too late. "By the time kids are 5 years old, the horse is out of the barn," says Dr. Leann L. Birch of the University of Georgia, an international authority on childhood obesity. That's why our book focuses on infancy.

Researchers now know that over 75 percent of obese eighth graders will remain obese into young adulthood and face a lifetime of struggle with their weight. One issue not often discussed is how obese children feel about their weight as they get older.

Dr. Robert Pretlow, a pediatrician, has collected online comments from many children who are obese. Here is a sample of what fifth and sixth graders had to say:

> "...I am 11 years old and I weigh 200–210 pounds. I need help. I am too embarrassed to consult my mom or dad about this... Depressed and embarrassed carl."

> "IM FAT! .... I DO NOT FIT IN THE desk AT SCHOOL! SO I HAVE TO SIT ALONE AT A TABLE!" BROOKE, AGE 11, Ht. 5'7", current 265 lb.

"... i weigh 267 ... my nicknames r hipo, elephant, floor crusher, fatty patty, giant gut, massive, chubs and more names that depress me"
patty, age 12

We don't want this to happen to your child. You may think these weight problems would never happen to your beautiful new baby. Yet recent data show that the risk is real. This book explains that what occurs during infancy can affect whether your baby becomes an overweight or obese kindergartner and remains that way through the years. In this book, we focus on the factors you *can* control during infancy to reduce the risk of obesity as your child grows older.

The infancy topics we discuss were chosen because there's evidence that each is linked to childhood obesity or its prevention. These topics include:

- Breastfeeding versus bottle feeding
- Overfeeding
- Rapid weight gain
- Sugar-sweetened beverages
- Sleep
- TV time
- Physical activity and outdoor play

Obesity tends to run in families and one of the reasons for this may be our genes. Some children inherit genes from their parents that may put them at greater risk of gaining excess weight. We can't change our genes, but we can control the genetic expression, or activity, of our genes to make it less likely that conditions such as type 2 diabetes and obesity will occur.

For example, research shows that eating a healthful diet, maintaining a healthy body weight and getting plenty of exercise can help turn off the expression of genes linked to type 2 diabetes. Similarly, researchers are finding that eating healthfully, exercising, reducing stress and nurturing a child can help turn off the expression of genes linked to obesity.

These lifestyle factors are discussed in this book since taking positive steps during infancy can help a child stay at a healthy weight, even if obesity seems to run in the family.

You probably know that during infancy, proper nutrition, plenty of sleep, fresh air, and regular check-ups are very important to your baby's future health. Yet, you may be bombarded with advice from family and friends, some of it conflicting and not backed by the latest scientific thinking. That makes it easy to feel overwhelmed and confused, and question whether you're doing what's best for your baby.

There's so much to consider—whether to breastfeed or bottle feed, when to start weaning, what to feed your baby and how to avoid overfeeding. Improper infant-feeding practices can lead to obesity, iron deficiency and other health problems for babies. We want to guide you toward making decisions that are good for your child's weight and health.

We'll explain how certain feeding practices can raise the risk of childhood obesity in ways you may not know. We'll delve into areas that have a bearing on childhood obesity, including a baby's rapid weight gain, sleep patterns, and physical activity, and we'll discuss special topics such as mothers who had weight-loss surgery, the impact of stress, and the role of grandparents.

Evidence suggests that infancy is one of the best times to prevent childhood obesity from developing. Our job is to inform you about how to help your child be at a healthy weight; your job is to make the choices that are best for you and your family.

Since we realize that not everyone will read all parts of this book, we included a glossary with definitions of useful terms. We also bolded some of the key messages in highlight boxes. Look for these important points throughout the book to help you and your child eat wisely, keep active and stay at a healthy weight.

Here's to a lifetime of good health and happiness for you and your family!

CHAPTER 1

Baby's First Food—It's Much More Than Milk

To prevent childhood obesity, the best way to feed an infant during the first year of life is to breastfeed. Breast milk is the closest thing we know to a miracle food. Here's why:

- It meets all the baby's nutritional needs (except for vitamin D and iron) for the first six months of life.
- It contains antibodies that protect a baby against viral and bacterial infections and reduce the need for antibiotics.
- It contains hormones and other growth factors that help the baby's gut to develop.
- It contains newly discovered hormones that influence the developing brain centers that control food intake and body weight.
- It's linked to higher intelligence when breastfeeding is continued for at least six months.
- **It plays an important role in preventing childhood obesity.**

Most of the pediatricians in America belong to the American Academy of Pediatrics (AAP) and look to it for guidance. The AAP recommends exclusive breastfeeding—feeding *only* breast milk—for at least six months. They say there's no doubt that breastfeeding protects babies against illnesses such as diarrhea, bacterial infections, diabetes, and childhood overweight and obesity. In addition to containing antibodies, there's evidence that breast milk helps to build the baby's own immune system, which protects him from disease.

From a mom's perspective, breastfeeding burns a lot of calories and causes the uterus to shrink. This helps her get back to her prepregnancy weight and shape, which is so important for preventing childhood obesity in future pregnancies.

But not everyone can breastfeed. Commercial formulas are very useful in special circumstances, such as when the mom is ill or the baby has medical problems that require a special formula diet. Moms may also choose to use infant formula because they find it more practical.

Although infant formulas have fewer health benefits than breast milk, formula can provide the calories and nutrients a growing baby needs. If formula feeding is the best choice for you, no worries. You shouldn't feel guilty about your decision, as babies do just fine on formula. Whether you breastfeed or formula feed, there's plenty of information in this book to help you keep your baby at a healthy weight.

The Gut-Brain Partnership: How It Affects Your Baby's Appetite and Weight

During pregnancy and the first year of life, a baby's brain develops very quickly—so quickly that his head rapidly increases in size. Breast milk provides exactly what's needed for a baby's developing brain, including the parts of the brain and nervous system that control food intake.

The brain's appetite centers consist of the hunger and satiety centers. The hunger center lets the baby know when he's hungry and wants to eat. That's all good. But if the baby eats too much, it can make him too fat. So a different part of the brain—the satiety center—lets the baby know that he's full and should stop eating. This system involves communication between the baby's gut—meaning the pancreas, stomach, liver, intestines, and fat tissue—and the baby's brain. If this gut-brain partnership works properly, the baby will eat enough food to meet his needs for growth and development, but not so much that he becomes fat.

Some body fat is healthy for babies. But too much fat, or obesity, is not healthy. Good communication between the infant gut and the appetite centers in the brain can help prevent childhood obesity by controlling how often and how much the baby eats.

The gut-brain partnership is a system in which the gut "talks" to the brain using nutrient, hormonal and nerve signals that tell whether the baby is hungry or not. The pictures on the following pages show how it works.

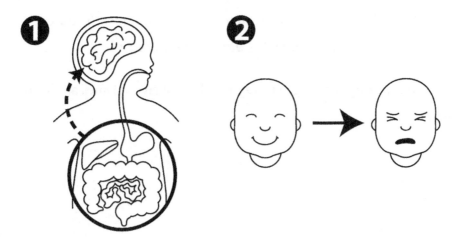

Figure 1: Several hours after a meal, the baby's stomach is empty. The gut signals the brain that hunger is developing (1). Appetite centers in the brain receive these signals and cause the baby's behavior to change (2).

For example, the baby might suck on his hand or get a bit fussy or cranky to signal that he's hungry. Babies use many different behaviors to signal hunger. For more information, see "Show Me the Signs" on page 33.

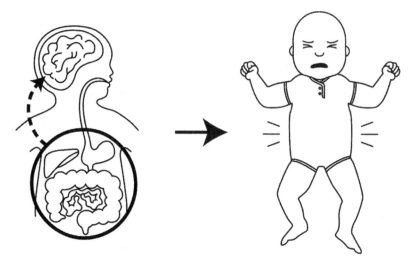

Figure 2: Once the baby feels hungry, the brain's appetite centers change his behavior. It's this changed behavior that lets the parent or caregiver know the baby needs to be fed.

Now it's up to the caregiver to recognize the baby's behavioral cues and respond appropriately.

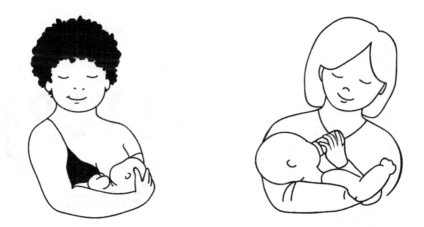

Figure 3: The mother or caregiver responds by feeding the baby.

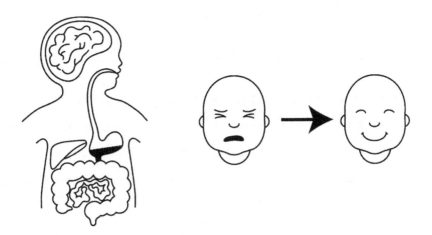

Figure 4: As feeding continues, nutrients are absorbed by the gut. The gut signals the brain that satiety (a feeling of fullness) is developing. The baby's feeding slows down and he will not suck as vigorously.

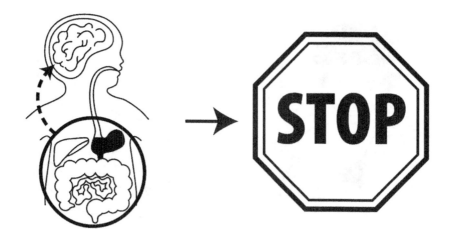

Figure 5: Once satiety is reached, the brain directs a further change in the baby's behavior. He stops feeding and, depending on his age, may turn his head away.

At this point, the meal ends. Satiety prevents further eating until hunger returns.

The problem is that the baby isn't always in charge of when to stop. He may be coaxed to continue feeding if the parent or caregiver doesn't realize that satiety has been reached and the meal should be over. Not respecting the baby's satiety signals and continuing to feed results in overfeeding, and this can lead to obesity.

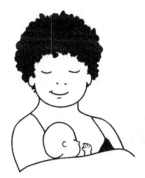 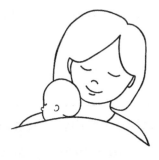

Figure 6: This is what it's like when the baby has had enough. Hunger is far away. Everyone's happy.

In summary, hunger and satiety are the two key factors in the gut-brain partnership that control how often and how much a baby eats. The baby's behavior will show you if he's hungry or if he's had enough. To put the baby in charge of his eating, it's important to learn how to read the cues. Correctly interpreting these cues will help you avoid overfeeding your baby.

For a bottle-fed baby, it may be tempting to coax him to finish what's left in the bottle. But to avoid overfeeding, it's more important to respect the baby's behavioral cues that he's had enough.

Whether you bottle-feed or breastfeed your baby, responding appropriately to these cues helps your baby learn to rely on his internal signals of hunger and satiety.

Recognizing and responding appropriately to these cues is very important to prevent obesity as he grows older.

A new mom brought her one-week-old to his first doctor visit. "Dr. Eden, how can I tell if my baby is eating enough?"

I answered, "Trust your baby. When he stops sucking vigorously, he is telling you he is done. Your baby should decide when the feeding is over. Your job is to tune in to your baby's signs that the meal should end."

Trust the baby when feeding. Baby knows best when he's hungry and when he's had enough.

Appetite Centers Develop Quickly During Infancy

The brain's appetite centers, which are the "brain half" of the gut-brain partnership, begin to develop almost from the moment pregnancy begins. The "gut half" starts to develop soon after. The flavors from the food mom eats travel into the amniotic fluid. During the last half of pregnancy, the baby swallows the flavorful fluid, which begins to shape his taste preferences.

That means if a mom chooses a variety of healthful foods before her baby's born, the developing baby gets exposed to the flavors of these foods. This pre-birth exposure to flavors influences the tastes the baby will learn to prefer after birth.

The gut-brain partnership must be ready to function as soon as the baby's born. This partnership continues to form during infancy and is influenced by your and your baby's diet. Having a well-developed gut-brain partnership during infancy means that when your child becomes a toddler and starts to take control of his own eating, he will be better able to regulate how much, how often and what he eats. By the time your preschooler's ready for kindergarten, the appetite centers of your child's brain are already set.

Leptin—A Hormone Messenger in the Gut-Brain Partnership

In the late 1990s, scientists were amazed to learn of a young girl who was normal weight at birth but started gaining weight very rapidly at 4 months old. As she aged, she was constantly hungry, demanded food all the time, and was very disruptive when she didn't receive it. By 9 years old, she was severely obese and weighed over 200 pounds.

It was discovered that this child lacked a special hormone called leptin. This hormone signals satiety and prompts a person to stop eating. When the child was given the leptin she lacked, her appetite rapidly returned to normal, as did her weight. The successful treatment of this rare case of obesity was the first clear evidence that leptin plays a key role in controlling appetite and how much we eat.

One important way that the infant gut communicates with the brain is through this hormone messenger, leptin. Scientists now know that leptin is found in the mother's colostrum—the fluid secreted by the mother's breasts in the first week of the baby's life—and also in breast milk.

A baby receives leptin when he drinks his mother's milk. The leptin gets absorbed in the baby's gut, and then travels through the bloodstream to the infant's brain. Here, leptin helps develop the brain regions that control appetite and feeding, and it signals mealtime satiety so that eating stops. Leptin isn't found in infant formula or foods commonly fed to infants.

It's likely that the leptin in the breast milk protected the little girl until 4 months old, an age when weaning from breast milk to solid foods often starts. The presence of leptin in colostrum and breast milk is a key benefit of breastfeeding. Leptin's role in controlling appetite and body weight strengthens our support for breastfeeding as one way to help prevent childhood obesity.

Breast Milk Helps Your Baby Feel Full

When a baby is breastfed, the composition of breast milk changes during the meal. This difference helps the baby know when he's had enough to eat. Foremilk is the breast milk produced at the start of a feeding. It's lower in fat but higher in protein and carbohydrate than hindmilk, or the milk produced at the end of a feeding. Hindmilk has more fat than foremilk. That's important since fat is a dietary signal that triggers satiety in the baby's brain.

Satiety is the opposite of hunger. This feeling of fullness develops slowly as the feeding progresses. But once satiety sets in, the baby's behavior will change. He will no longer suck vigorously and may even get annoyed if coaxed to eat. His behavior means he's had enough and the feeding is over.

The hormones in breast milk also differ at the start and the end of the meal. Ghrelin is a hunger hormone, so ghrelin levels are higher in foremilk, when the baby starts to feed, than in hindmilk, when the baby's not as hungry. Leptin is a satiety hormone, so leptin levels start out low in foremilk and increase as the breast milk changes to hindmilk. Leptin signals the end of the meal and feeding stops.

The Flavors of Breast Milk Shape Your Baby's Tastes

Your baby's gut-brain partnership is affected by the food choices you make. If you choose to breastfeed, the flavors from the foods and drinks you consume will make their way into your breast milk, and your baby will taste these flavors when she drinks your milk.

Dr. Julie Mennella, a researcher at Monell Chemical Senses Center in Philadelphia, has shown that babies exposed to the flavors of fruits and vegetables during breastfeeding are more willing to accept these foods once they start eating solids.

A new mom was eager to get an answer to her question on vegetables. "Dr. Eden," she asked, "I love broccoli but not a lot of other vegetables. Is it OK if I eat broccoli almost every day?"

I replied, "Varying your vegetables is important for nutritional reasons, but if broccoli is one of the few vegetables that you like, then it's fine to eat it as often as you do. The foods you eat affect the flavors of your breast milk and that influences your baby's taste preferences. By eating broccoli, along with other vegetables, you're giving your baby a good start in liking vegetables."

Drinking alcoholic beverages, smoking, and eating sugary foods can also affect the flavors of breast milk. Blood alcohol levels rise after drinking, and when blood levels are high the alcohol passes into the breast milk. Studies show that if a baby's breastfed soon after mom has a drink, the baby tastes the alcohol. This causes him to drink less milk. There's also a concern that if mom drinks alcohol regularly and the baby keeps getting a taste of it when feeding, then the baby may prefer alcohol when he gets older. Since alcohol calories add up quickly when drinking, discouraging a preference for alcohol early on may help with weight control later in life.

If a mom smokes, the nicotine and chemicals from tobacco smoke enter her breast milk. This changes the flavor of the breast milk, which the baby tastes.

Sugary foods and drinks also affect the flavor of breast milk. Since taste preferences are being shaped during infancy, including the desire for sweet tastes, it's best if a breastfeeding mom quenches her thirst with water instead of juice or sugary drinks.

By making wise lifestyle choices, you'll give your baby a "taste" of wholesome habits and an early start to enjoying foods that are good for his health and his weight. For more information, see "Alcohol, Tobacco and Drugs" on page 105.

If mom eats fruits and vegetables, her baby will taste the flavors in her breast milk. This makes the baby more accepting of these foods when he starts eating solids.

The Good Gut Bacteria

Starting at birth, the infant gut houses bacteria that are good for your baby, as well as some that are not so good. The good gut bacteria benefit your baby's health; some may even help prevent obesity. The bad gut bacteria can't be avoided, but too many can make your baby sick.

Bruce German, a University of California scientist who studies breast milk and gut bacteria, says breast milk is the one thing that has evolved to protect babies against disease. That's because breast milk contains antibodies and other substances that support a proper balance between the good and bad bacteria. This balance affects the baby's immune system. Breast milk contains indigestible compounds that are there to feed the good bacteria in the baby's gut. Since breast milk helps the healthy bacteria to grow, the bad gut bacteria have less of a chance of making the baby ill. As Dr. German says, "It's as important to feed the bacteria in the baby as the baby."

Breastfeeding is the ideal way for the baby to have a healthy balance of gut bacteria. Infant formula doesn't match all the health-promoting properties of breast milk. However, research is currently under way to improve the composition of infant formula so that it more closely mimics breast milk in supporting the growth of good bacteria.

Gut Bacteria, Antibiotics and Obesity

Recent studies suggest that the balance of good and bad gut bacteria may help prevent obesity. Researchers found that mice given gut bacteria from obese humans got fat, while mice given gut bacteria from lean humans did not get fat. Studies have also shown that the most common bacteria in people who are obese are different from the most common bacteria in people who are lean. Researchers continue to explore the connection between gut bacteria and obesity.

It's believed that antibiotic use in babies may increase the risk of obesity. Consider that for decades, farmers have been feeding antibiotics—drugs that kill gut bacteria—to animals such as cows, pigs and chickens, to make them grow faster and fatter.

Antibiotics change the healthy balance of good and bad bacteria in the gut. Evidence shows that breastfed babies have stronger immune protection and use fewer antibiotics than formula-fed babies. This may help protect breastfed babies from developing childhood obesity.

Breastfeeding isn't a guarantee against illness or obesity. Whether you breastfeed or bottle feed your baby, try to use antibiotics only when necessary to minimize the effect on good gut bacteria. But do take antibiotics when needed, such as for certain bacterial illnesses. If you have any concerns, speak with your child's pediatrician.

How Feeding Style is Linked to Childhood Obesity

Whether you breastfeed or bottle feed, you have a choice of how to feed your baby—on demand or on a schedule. Did you know that one feeding style may protect against childhood obesity more than the other?

Demand feeding, also called responsive feeding, means that you feed your baby only when his behavior signals that he's hungry and wants to eat. Scheduled feeding means that you feed your baby on a set schedule, about the same times every day. A large study of American children followed from birth to kindergarten suggests that demand feeding during infancy protects against childhood obesity.

During infancy, the gut-brain partnership that controls eating develops rapidly. Demand feeding responds to the internal feelings of hunger. He may start to fuss or cry, and that's your cue that he needs to be fed. A baby fed on a set schedule may not be hungry at mealtime.

Demand feeding allows you to identify and respond appropriately to your baby's behavioral cues. Since he can't talk, these cues are the only way he communicates that he's hungry.

Demand feeding is desirable for both breastfed and bottle-fed babies. To protect against childhood obesity, we recommend demand feeding, although we realize that for some moms it may be more practical to have a set schedule for feeding.

If others are assisting with your baby's feeding, help them to recognize your baby's hunger and satiety cues.

This will let them know when your baby needs to be fed and when he's full and is finished feeding. Respecting the baby's satiety cues will help prevent overfeeding.

Crying can mean many things, but studies show that it can lead to overfeeding. Aim to feed your baby when he's truly hungry and avoid using food as a way to soothe an upset child. To better understand your baby's cry, see "Is a Crying Baby a Hungry Baby?" on page 49.

Show Me the Signs

Your baby's behavior is your cue for when he's hungry and when he's full. If you pay close attention, his behavior will tell you what he wants before he starts to cry.

Signs That Your Baby is Hungry

Not all babies use the same signs, but your baby may use some of these:

- **Rooting for the breast.** A breastfed baby will move his head from side to side looking for the breast. This movement is instinctual and is called the rooting reflex. If your baby hasn't eaten in a few hours, while you're sitting back at a comfortable angle, place your baby upright and hold him against your skin between your breasts. If your baby's hungry, you'll likely see the rooting reflex.

- **Movements of his mouth, lips or tongue that suggest feeding.** Your baby may open and close his mouth as if he's trying to latch on to the nipple. He may stick out his tongue or make sucking motions with his mouth.

- **Hand to mouth action.** Your baby may put his hand, a piece of clothing, or a blanket into his mouth and start sucking on it.

- **Increased alertness.** You may notice that he's more aware of a light touch on one side of his face and he will turn his head and move toward the touch looking for something to suck on.

Premature babies and babies less than 6 weeks old will need small feedings of breast milk or formula quite often. It's not unusual to feed such young babies eight to twelve times a day. Whether you breastfeed or bottle feed your baby, try using skin-to-skin contact to help you "tune-in" to your baby's signals. Studies show that skin-to-skin contact promotes successful breastfeeding, possibly by helping you respond to your baby's feeding cues.

Signs That Your Baby is Full

If your baby does any of these things after feeding, it's a sign that he's had enough:

- Sucks less vigorously
- Becomes sleepy
- Loses interest or gets annoyed if you try to continue feeding
- Turns his head or body to signal he's full (in older babies)

When your baby shows that he's had enough, don't coax him to drink more. To help prevent obesity, if you're using a bottle to feed him expressed breast milk or formula and there's only a small amount left, it's better to honor your baby's satiety signals and discard the rest.

Keep in mind that some babies like to feed and sleep more than others. Babies grow rapidly during the first year of life. But they don't grow at a constant rate; they grow in spurts. The desire to feed and sleep are usually greater during growth spurts and will subside when growth slows down. The challenge is to trust your baby. He knows when he's hungry and when he's full.

CHAPTER 2

Breastfeeding or Bottle Feeding–What's Your Choice?

How do you want to feed your baby—by breast or with formula? From a childhood obesity perspective, there's evidence that breastfeeding may offer more protection against obesity later in life. However, you might feel that bottle feeding with formula is the right choice. If you haven't decided yet, here's what you need to know to inform your decision and minimize the risk of your growing baby becoming an overweight child.

The Benefits of Breastfeeding

Partly because of the hormones in breast milk that regulate appetite, exclusive breastfeeding protects against childhood obesity. This is especially so if breast milk is the baby's only food for the first six months of life. After that, breastfeeding should ideally be continued, but solid foods can be introduced, one at a time.

According to the Centers for Disease Control and Prevention (CDC), a baby's risk of becoming obese decreases with each additional month of exclusive breastfeeding.

Exclusive breastfeeding means feeding your baby only breast milk for her first six months—that means no formula, juice, soda or pop, sugar water, honey, fruit drinks, or infant cereal by spoon or mixed with milk in a bottle. Even water isn't needed, although after 2 months old a little bit is OK on a hot day. Babies under

12 months old should never be fed honey since it may contain dangerous spores that can grow in the baby's intestinal tract and cause fatal infant botulism.

However, breastfed babies do need vitamin D starting when they're a few days old. Check with your baby's pediatrician for guidance.

Here's what the American Academy of Pediatrics (AAP) has to say about breastfeeding:

> *The American Academy of Pediatrics recommends exclusive breastfeeding for the first six months, followed by continued breastfeeding as complementary foods are introduced, with continuation of breastfeeding for one year or longer as mutually desired by mother and infant.*

Following this AAP recommendation is the most important thing you can do in the first year of your baby's life to prevent childhood obesity. If you've returned to work or are unable to breastfeed as often as you'd like, consider pumping your milk so that a caregiver can feed the baby breast milk from a bottle in your absence. If you choose to bottle feed, be aware of your baby's hunger and satiety cues, and avoid overfeeding once your baby shows signs that she's full. This will help prevent future obesity.

The American Academy of Pediatrics recommends six months of exclusive breastfeeding.

Breastfeeding also benefits a mom. Breastfeeding:

- Helps your uterus to contract, so you can return to your pre-pregnancy tummy tone, weight and shape more quickly.

- Responds to the increasing demands of your growing baby. The longer breastfeeding continues and the more your baby grows, the more milk she will need and the more calories you'll use to support milk production.

- Burns a whopping 800 calories per day by the time your baby's about 4 months old. This large calorie burn can help you lose the extra weight gained while pregnant.

- **Helps prevent childhood obesity if you become pregnant again.** Reaching a healthy weight before getting pregnant is important, since the number one predictor of childhood obesity is maternal obesity (a body mass index [BMI] of 30 or higher). To check your BMI visit the Shape Up America!® website at *www.shapeup.org* and select "BMI calculator" from the Adults menu.

- Helps prevent breast and ovarian cancer.

While discussing the benefits of breastfeeding, 19-year-old Rebecca cringed. "But Dr. Eden, I was told by my friend that breastfeeding will cause my breasts to sag, and I don't want that to happen."

I responded, "No worries; that's simply not true. Most moms find that their breasts go back to their prepregnancy shape and size after they stop breastfeeding. Aging, gravity and gaining weight may change the shape of your breasts, but that will not happen because of breastfeeding."

As wonderful as breastfeeding is, it takes getting used to. Learning the proper technique, practicing, and having support from family and friends will help make it easier. If you have twins or a premature baby, you can still breastfeed, if you so choose. It's best to seek guidance from a breastfeeding specialist. For more information on breastfeeding and finding a lactation consultant, see Appendix B.

Is Your Hospital Baby-friendly?

A baby-friendly hospital supports breastfeeding and is awarded that name only if it meets 10 specific criteria for promoting breastfeeding. According to Baby-Friendly USA, there are currently 187 U.S. hospitals and birthing centers across the country that are designated baby-friendly. The number of such hospitals is increasing, from 2.9 percent of U.S. babies born in baby-friendly facilities in 2007 to 7.7 percent in 2014. If you're reading this book before giving birth and would like to breastfeed, you can find out if there's a baby-friendly hospital near you at *www.babyfriendlyusa.org/find-facilities*.

Most women in the U.S. choose to breastfeed for at least the first few weeks after giving birth. But very few of these moms are still breastfeeding after three or four months. Both the World Health Organization (WHO) and the Centers for Disease Control and Prevention (CDC) want hospitals to do more to support breastfeeding. Both organizations support the adoption of *Ten Steps to Successful Breastfeeding*. Hospitals must adhere to all of these steps if they want to be called "baby-friendly." These steps include helping moms to begin breastfeeding within one hour of giving birth, showing moms how to breastfeed, practicing rooming-in (see below) and encouraging breastfeeding on demand.

According to a 2013 study, there are four practices that together are strongly linked to **successful breastfeeding**:

- Initiating breastfeeding within the first hour after giving birth
- Having skin-to-skin contact between mom and baby
- Rooming-in
- No supplementing breastfeeding with formula while in the hospital

Yet, most hospitals don't help moms initiate breastfeeding within one hour after giving birth. And too many hospitals undermine successful breastfeeding by allowing mom to supplement breast milk with formula even before she and her newborn are used to breastfeeding. In one national survey of infant feeding practices, 42 percent of babies were fed formula supplements while in the hospital. In a 2011 survey published by the CDC, only 1 out of 5 hospitals had a written policy limiting the use of formula supplements for breastfeeding moms. Feeding a newborn formula supplements is known to undermine breastfeeding.

Baby-friendly hospitals help moms learn how to breastfeed successfully. A new mom needs to learn how to help her baby latch on to her breast. This latching-on process is often more difficult for an obese mom or someone with inverted nipples, so she may need additional support to do it properly. A mom also needs to understand how to position her baby to encourage latching on. If your hospital isn't baby-friendly or you need additional guidance, reassurance or problem-solving support, contact a certified lactation consultant or check out the International Lactation Consultant Association at *www.ilca.org*.

Rooming-in allows a mom and her baby to remain together 24 hours a day. Many hospitals don't support rooming-in, but baby-friendly hospitals encourage this practice. In the first few days after birth, a breastfed baby will need to feed about eight to twelve times every 24 hours. Healthy babies should be allowed to develop their own feeding schedules and not have to follow the hospital's schedule. Rooming-in makes feeding easier because it allows you to listen to your baby and learn to recognize the signs that she is ready to eat.

Whether you breastfeed or formula feed, rooming-in lets you bond with your baby and learn how to feed on demand. Bonding and demand, or responsive, feeding can help you avoid overfeeding and the possibility of your child gaining excessive weight as she gets older.

If the hospital near you doesn't qualify for the designation "baby friendly" and you're reading this book before your baby's born, you can still discuss these issues with your doctor. Let your doctor know that you want to breastfeed and explain what your wishes are.

Breastfeeding Saves Money

One of the many benefits of breastfeeding is that it costs less than formula feeding. An analysis from 2007 estimated that one year of infant formula costs over $1,700, not including bottles, nipples or bottled water, which some parents prefer to use. The cost could be even more if a special formula is needed.

When a newborn is eating tiny amounts of formula, the cost may not seem like much. But as a baby grows and drinks more formula, the cost also grows. According to one survey conducted by the CDC, some moms admitted that to cut the cost of formula, they introduced solid foods as early as four weeks and the majority started before the baby was four months old. The AAP recognizes there is no need to wean a baby before six months. Introducing solid foods too early increases the risk of childhood obesity.

If costs are a concern, keep in mind that breastfeeding is cheaper and more convenient than formula feeding. There are no bottles to warm and clean. Plus it's an emotionally beneficial experience. Holding your baby close to your heart when breastfeeding lets you bond with your baby, reduces stress in mom and baby, and helps your baby feel secure. Studies show that maternal-infant bonding and feeling less stressed may help prevent childhood obesity.

Babies Lose Weight the First Week of Life

Don't worry if your baby loses weight in her first week. During pregnancy, babies grow while floating in the fluid-filled amniotic sac. Babies "dry out" during the first week of life and the water loss causes weight loss even when the baby's fed well. That happens whether your baby is fed colostrum, which is the breast milk produced right after birth, or infant formula. This first-week weight loss, which could be up to 10 percent of your baby's birth weight, is normal and isn't a cause for concern.

If you chose to breastfeed, know that despite this early weight loss, you're still likely producing enough breast milk to feed your baby. So don't let this early weight loss discourage you from breastfeeding.

Is it OK to Stop Breastfeeding Early?

We recommend that moms breastfeed exclusively for at least six months, and then continue to breastfeed while introducing solid foods. That may not be practical for all moms. Perhaps you have to return to work, or you become ill, or you just want to take a temporary break from breastfeeding. The good news is that you can still feed your baby breast milk by expressing your breast milk by hand or by using a manual or electric pump. You can pump breast milk and store it in the refrigerator to use later on or the following day. Or you can freeze it. An added benefit of pumping and storing milk is that it lets the baby's dad or caregivers bond with the baby while bottle feeding her with your breast milk.

However, if pumping milk isn't what you had in mind, you could use supplementary feedings of commercial infant formula. Infants quickly learn to accept both the breast and a bottle.

Helpful Tips for Bottle Feeding

While breastfeeding is best, it's not for everyone. Breastfeeding isn't advised for moms who have certain infectious or chronic diseases, use illegal drugs, or take some medications (although most prescription drugs are fine). For these women, it's best to follow their doctor's advice.

If you're thinking about bottle feeding, here are some points to consider:

- Nutritionally, infant formula comes close to breast milk. Although formula doesn't have the infection-fighting antibodies and appetite-regulating hormones found in breast milk, it does provide the nutrients your baby needs for proper growth and development.

- You can form a loving bond with your bottle-fed baby. Hold your baby close—skin-to-skin when possible—talk to her, and enjoy the time spent together while she feeds.

- You can avoid overfeeding by tuning in to your baby's satiety cues. This will help prevent your child from becoming overweight. See "Show Me the Signs" on page 33.

- If you choose to bottle feed your baby, it's still important that you eat healthfully. It's not too early to be a good role model for your growing child. Someday soon she'll notice the foods you're eating and start to reach for them and put them in her mouth. So let the foods she reaches for be healthful.

If you can't or choose not to breastfeed, don't feel guilty about using formula. Follow the tips on bottle feeding in this chapter to help your baby feed well and be healthy.

Bottle-feeding With Formula or Expressed Breast Milk

You can bottle feed a baby using infant formula or expressed breast milk. Try these tips to get the most out of bottle feeding your baby:

- Bottle feeding is a good time to bond with your baby. Cuddle her, smile at her, talk to her. Don't prop the bottle and leave her alone to feed herself. Instead, take advantage of this special time to bond with your baby.

- Share bonding time with your spouse or partner. Take a short break and let others who care for your baby feed her and enjoy the time together.

- Help your baby swallow properly by holding her upright in your arms. Make sure she drinks from a bottle angled down so that milk fills the nipple and she isn't sucking in air.

- Avoid placing a bottle in your baby's mouth and propping it against a pillow to hold it in place. Teething babies who suck on a bottle of milk, juice or sugar water while lying down can develop "nursing bottle" caries or tooth decay. If your baby needs something to suck on to fall asleep, try a pacifier.

- Remember that you're shaping your baby's taste preferences. Avoid early exposure to foods and drinks with added sugar. This will help your baby learn to prefer unsweetened varieties. It will also help prevent tooth decay and excess weight gain now and later on.

Bottle-prep Safety

For safety's sake, once you prepare a bottle for your baby, use it within one hour. Then discard the contents so it doesn't get contaminated with bacteria. Breast milk that is expressed and put into a bottle can also grow bacteria. It should be kept refrigerated until it's needed, but even if refrigerated, use it within four days or discard it. Once it has reached room temperature, it should be discarded after six hours.

Never use a microwave to heat a bottle. Since a microwave heats unevenly, it's possible that the hot spots could burn the baby's mouth. To warm a bottle, place it in a bowl of hot water for just a few minutes. To make sure the liquid isn't too hot, turn the bottle upside down a few times so the liquid is mixed well. Then test the liquid on the inside of your wrist before feeding your baby. It should feel slightly warm but not hot.

Iron Rules When Switching from Breastfeeding to Formula

Breastfed babies need additional iron from the time they're about 4 months old. Iron is important for your baby's brain development and it prevents iron deficiency anemia. We recommend an iron-fortified vitamin supplement, but check with your pediatrician.

If you started out breastfeeding and want to switch to bottle feeding before your baby's 1 year old, be sure to use an iron-fortified formula. By the time your breastfed baby is 6 months old, most of the iron she received from you during pregnancy will have been depleted. Baby cereals are fortified with iron in a form that's well absorbed. This helps replenish the baby's iron stores.

If your baby's been fed formula from birth, continue to give her formula until she turns one. Whether you started out breastfeeding or formula feeding, don't switch to regular cow's milk. Cow's milk contains practically no iron. Giving it to your baby during her first year of life will lead to iron deficiency. Since iron deficiency may be associated with learning disabilities later on, it's essential that you prevent it now. After your baby's first birthday, it's OK to switch to full-fat (whole) cow's milk.

Do not give your baby cow's milk until she has reached her first birthday.

You can start to introduce solid foods at 6 months old. Include iron-rich foods, such as infant cereal, egg, and pureed or strained meats and green vegetables.

It's important that your baby gets all the nutrients she needs for growth and development. There's evidence that iron, along with zinc, folic acid and vitamin B_{12}, are especially important for the development of the gut-brain partnership. See "The Gut-Brain Partnership: How It Affects Your Baby's Appetite and Weight" on page 20.

Chapter 3

How to Help Your Baby Stay at a Healthy Weight

Growing babies don't have to become obese children. Whether you breastfeed or bottle feed, these strategies can prevent your child from gaining too much weight.

Your Number One Goal: Avoid Overfeeding

A newborn has a very small stomach. How small? Make a circle by tucking your forefinger into the base of your thumb. That little circle is about the size of a newborn's stomach. It doesn't take much milk for your baby's tummy to feel full—about 1 to 1.5 teaspoons will be enough. By the end of the first week, your baby's tummy will increase to about the size of a walnut and will hold about 1.5 to 2 ounces—still pretty small!

Regardless of whether you breastfeed or bottle feed, the challenge is to avoid overfeeding by tuning in to your baby's behavior—the cues that signal either hunger or satiety.

Overfeeding a baby can lead to childhood obesity. It can happen if you:

- Don't recognize when your baby's full and feeding is over
- Coax your baby to eat too much and too often

Bottle-fed babies are more likely to be overfed than breastfed babies. That's because it's easy to see how much was in the bottle to start and how much is left when the baby shows signs that he's had enough. The cost of formula may tempt parents to keep feeding their baby so the formula isn't wasted. But feeding to the last drop means the baby's satiety cues are ignored and the baby isn't able to decide for himself when the meal's over.

On the other hand, breasts are not marked off in ounces. A breastfeeding mom has no way of knowing how much her baby has consumed. Feeding is likely to stop when the baby decides he doesn't want more.

There's some evidence that bottle-fed babies may have less control over how much they eat than breastfed babies. As a result, they may gain weight more quickly than breastfed babies. For example, one study found that babies who were bottle fed through 6 months old were twice as likely as babies who were breastfed to drink everything in a bottle or cup when they were over 6 months old. This may indicate that the satiety signals in the bottle-fed babies were not effective.

In another study, babies were divided into three groups: breastfed only, bottle fed only and a combination of breastfed and bottle fed. When the BMI of the babies at month 5 was compared to their BMI at month 2, the bottle fed babies increased their BMI by 14.6 percent, while the breastfed babies increased by only 3.5 percent. The increase in BMI in the babies that were combination fed was in-between, at 11.8 percent.

What to do? Whether you bottle feed or breastfeed, it's important to recognize the signs that your baby has had enough to eat and to stop feeding. This will prevent overfeeding and help your baby learn to self-regulate his eating. This self-regulation will continue as he gets older and can help prevent obesity later in life. See "Show Me the Signs" on page 33.

Is a Crying Baby a Hungry Baby?

New parents may think that when a baby cries, it's because he's hungry and wants food. That's not always the case and could lead to overfeeding. In fact, some studies suggest that overfeeding is linked to not understanding the reasons a baby cries.

A baby cries for many reasons besides being hungry. A crying baby may:

- Feel lonely
- Be tired
- Want attention
- Need a diaper change
- Want a hug
- Feel gassy

How do you know if it's a cry for food or something else? After a baby is a couple of weeks old, it takes at least three hours for his stomach to empty after a feeding. So if your baby's crying only one hour after feeding, it's unlikely to be from hunger.

If your baby cries, it may be for a reason that's not about food. Perhaps he's cranky because he didn't get enough physical activity during the day to tire him out, so he didn't want to go to sleep. Or perhaps he just wants to interact with you. Some parents learn to detect what a baby's cry means because the various cries may sound different. For example, some moms can hear the different sounds of a tired cry, hungry cry, frustrated cry, or a something hurts cry.

When your baby cries, first try to hold or rock him to quiet his fussing. Then give some thought to what may be prompting him to cry. It's possible that it's something other than being hungry.

> *One evening at 1:00 a.m., a new mom called. She said, "Dr. Eden, my 3-week-old little boy is crying and I just fed him. What should I do?"*
>
> *I answered, "You know that your baby cannot email or text you; all he can do is cry. Crying is a baby's first language and it's up to you as a parent to figure out why. A cry from hunger is different than a cry from being sleepy or needing a diaper change. You will get a better idea of what the different cries sound like and what they mean over the next couple of weeks."*

Whatever the reason a baby cries at night, sleep is important for everyone and may help prevent obesity in you and your child. See "Lack of Sleep—A Link to Childhood Obesity" on page 73.

Some Tips for Comforting Your Baby

Here are some **non-food** ways to comfort and soothe your crying baby:

- Give your baby a warm bath to see if that calms him down.
- Have your baby listen to or watch running water.
- Gently swing your baby in a baby-swing.
- Hold your baby in your arms and rock him in a rocking chair.
- Lay your baby tummy-down across your lap and gently pat or rub his back.
- Run the vacuum cleaner or a fan that makes "white noise."

- Give your baby something new to look at or hold.

- Take your baby outside for some fresh air.

- Take your baby for a ride in a car.

- Go for a walk with your baby in a stroller; you'll get some exercise and a release of frustration, too.

If you've tried everything, ask for help from family or friends. Don't wait until you're seriously sleep deprived to get assistance. Besides making it harder to think straight, lack of sleep may increase the risk of obesity in adults.

Timmy was a 2-month-old who had colic. He cried and cried. It seemed like the only way he could be soothed was by strapping him into his car seat and driving him around the neighborhood. The problem was that Timmy was at his worst at 2:00 a.m. Timmy's mom said, "Dr. Eden, one time when I was driving, we were pulled over by the police. The officer was suspicious of a car driving slowly around the block. But the driving helped my baby to calm down and go to sleep."

A Love Connection—How to Bond with Your Baby

Breastfeeding creates a deep bond between a mom and her baby. If you breastfeed, this bond starts as soon as you begin feeding, which ideally should be within the first hour of giving birth. The CDC recommends that, for the first few days, you breastfeed about eight to twelve times every 24 hours. Frequent feedings will help you make plenty of milk and give you many opportunities to bond with your baby.

Whether you breastfeed or bottle feed your baby, it's very important to encourage this special bond. Bonding calms and soothes both of you, as you develop your relationship with each other. Try to make skin-to-skin contact with your baby, with his skin touching your skin, as much as possible.

As you hold your baby when breastfeeding, special hormones are stimulated that encourage milk production and milk let-down—the milk ejection reflex—as well as parent-child bonding. If you bottle feed, hold your baby close, skin-to-skin, and this will stimulate the same hormones that promote a sense of bonding. You may find that your heartbeat soothes your baby.

A dad, grandparent or other caregiver also benefits from bonding with the baby. Hold the baby close to your heart while giving him a bottle. Forming a bond with your baby will bring joy and comfort to you and the baby.

> *Judy told a story about the special bond between her mom and newborn daughter Taylor. "Dr. Eden, when my daughter was born prematurely, I was so exhausted and not feeling very well that my wonderful mom came to help so I could get some sleep. She told me, 'I instinctively held my beautiful granddaughter Taylor on my chest when she was 2 days old. To quiet her, I held her close for a long time so she could hear my heartbeat. We have had a strong bond ever since.'"*

This special one-on-one time for caregivers other than mom is also important because it helps them tune in to the baby's cues that he's hungry or full. This is very important if they're going to share responsibility for feeding your baby.

CHAPTER 4

The Right Time for Solid Foods

No Need to Rush

The AAP recommends waiting until a baby's about 6 months old before introducing solid foods. Yet, a large percentage of babies are being fed solid foods much too early. One survey of 268 babies found that 57 percent of 2-month-olds were already eating infant cereal, and 87 percent were eating cereal at 3 months. Even more disturbing, in a recent survey conducted by the CDC, 2 out of 3 moms who introduced solid foods too early said they did so on the recommendation of a healthcare professional!

A few decades ago, it was quite common to start babies on solid foods when they were just a few weeks old. Now experts know that introducing solid foods too early isn't a good idea. Here's why:

- Until a baby is at least 4 months old, her digestive tract and gut bacteria have not developed enough to process solid foods, including cereal. Introducing solids too soon may cause diarrhea, bloody stools, vomiting and abdominal pain.

- Before 4 or 5 months old, a baby can hardly sit up or hold her head up properly. So feeding solid foods before then may lead to choking.

- If a baby is fed solid foods when just a couple of months old, she will not yet be able to turn away from a spoon when no longer interested in eating. This can lead to overfeeding.

- Introducing solid foods too early has been linked to obesity, diabetes, eczema and celiac disease.

Here are some signs that your baby's ready to try solid foods:

- She can sit up well.
- Her neck muscles are strong enough to hold her head up.
- She swallows well.
- She can keep milk in her mouth instead of letting it dribble.
- She's interested in what you're eating and may try to grab food from your plate.
- Her birth weight has doubled.

Babies vary in their readiness to accept solid foods. A bottle-fed baby who drinks more than a quart of formula each day and continually cries for more between feedings will need solid foods sooner than a baby who drinks less but is content between feedings. So watch for signs of readiness after 4 or 5 months old. If your baby has reached 6 months, is fussier between meals and wants more when the bottle is empty, it's time to start introducing solid foods. If your breastfed baby seems hungry even with longer or more frequent feedings, then that's a sign to supplement breastfeeding with solid foods.

Once your baby's ready for solids and has good control over her head and neck muscles, she'll be able to turn away when she's had enough to eat. Let your baby decide when she's done. Respecting your baby's signals to end a meal is one way to prevent overfeeding.

Getting Started on Solid Foods

When your baby's ready to include solid foods along with breast milk or formula, the transition to solid foods should be done carefully, as food choices and amounts can have long-lasting effects on your baby's health and weight.

Babies of the same age can develop at very different rates. This section provides some guidance on the approximate age to introduce solid foods. It will give you an idea of the foods that are typical first foods and when they're usually fed.

Starting on Solids

Age	Foods	When
6 months	Precooked infant cereals (mix with formula or expressed breast milk, not with cow's milk)	Breakfast and dinner
7 months	Cooked and strained single fruits or mashed raw fruit (fed without formula or expressed breast milk), such as strained apple and mashed banana	Breakfast and dinner
8 months	Cooked and strained vegetables (fed without formula or expressed breast milk), such as green beans, carrots, sweet potatoes	Lunch
8–9 months	Cooked egg yolk, low-sugar dry cereal such as original Cheerios® Small pieces of pasta	Breakfast Lunch or dinner
9 months	Cooked and strained meats, such as lean beef, chicken; cooked beans Plain yogurt	Lunch Snacks
10–12 months	Cottage cheese (preferably no-salt-added), teething biscuits, small pieces of fruit	Snacks

Foods should be introduced one at a time. Wait three to five days, or even a bit longer, before introducing the next food. That way, if your baby has a bad reaction to a food, you'll be able to identify the offending food and avoid it. Symptoms to look for include diarrhea, vomiting, skin rash, stomach pain, coughing, congestion, ear infection and being very irritable.

If the symptoms are severe, the food should be avoided entirely until the next appointment with your baby's pediatrician. At that appointment, be sure to discuss the problem and what the next steps should be.

Introduce only one food at a time. Wait three to five days before introducing the next food.

A new mom described an unsettling situation when her daughter Amanda did not want to eat anymore. "Dr. Eden," she said, "I'm worried. I remember telling my husband, 'Amanda just isn't eating enough!' " But visits to my office showed that Amanda was developing well and gaining weight at an appropriate rate. She clearly was eating enough.

I explained, "As long as your daughter is growing well, if she sometimes eats only a little at a meal, that's OK. Overfeeding can lead to obesity so you want to be careful not to coax your baby to eat too much and too often.

"Tuning in to Amanda's cues of when she's hungry and when she's had enough is very important. So is coming regularly to her doctor visits to have her growth rate checked. This will help make sure Amanda is eating nutritiously and getting enough for her growing needs."

Finger Foods for Babies

By about 9 months old, most babies will start to pick up small pieces of food and try to feed themselves. This gives babies some control over what and how much they eat. Here are some ideas for nutritious finger foods for your baby. Be sure to stay with her while she eats, to make sure she doesn't choke.

- Colorful chopped or sliced cooked veggies, such as carrots, broccoli, green beans or peas
- Veggie strips such as red pepper or zucchini strips with hummus
- Chopped, cooked sweet potato
- Diced avocado
- Chopped, soft fruit such as peaches, melon, mango, or canned fruit in juice (not syrup)
- Small pieces of banana, strawberries or blueberries
- Sliced kiwi
- Baked apple cubes or melon cubes dipped in plain full-fat yogurt or soy yogurt
- Dry, iron-fortified, low-sugar cereals such as original Cheerios®, Corn Chex® or Rice Chex®
- Pieces of whole-grain bread or strips of tortilla
- Baby crackers or teething biscuits
- Cooked whole-wheat pasta or tri-color pasta mixed with very small pieces of cooked ground meat or chicken
- Scrambled egg and cheese
- Tofu cubes
- Cooked black beans
- Sliced cheese

Babies Prefer Plain Foods

Babies have different taste preferences than adults, so what is tasty to you may not be so yummy to your baby. Babies are not necessarily born with a "sweet tooth." They learn to like sweets. If you feed your baby sugary or salty foods that you like to eat, you're exposing her to adult tastes that she may not prefer at this point. In fact, you may be encouraging sweet and salty preferences that can one day lead to overeating. Giving your baby sugary and salty foods changes the areas of her developing brain that influence taste preferences. A baby is fine with bland foods, although that will change soon enough.

> One afternoon the mother of 8-month-old Jenny called. She said, "Dr. Eden, I just tasted Jenny's lunch of plain, strained vegetables and it has absolutely no taste. Should I add some salt to give it more flavor?"

> I answered, "You don't have to add salt to Jenny's lunch. At this age, she will be content with bland-tasting food. Plus, she doesn't need the extra salt."

Sugar and Salt–An Unhealthy Duo

Wholesome foods like fruits and vegetables provide enough naturally-occurring sugar to meet your baby's needs. Too much sugar adds unnecessary calories and can lead to tooth decay once a baby's teeth start coming in.

Extra salt is also not necessary for a baby. The good news is that most commercial baby foods no longer have added salt and most don't have added sugar. But new products are introduced all the time, so check the ingredient list to be sure.

Remember that during infancy, you're shaping your baby's taste preferences. The aim is to keep your child at a healthy weight. If you give your baby foods or drinks with added sugar or salt, she'll soon prefer those tastes and continue to want sugary or salty foods as she grows.

Instead, offer your baby nutritious foods without added sugar and salt. For a sweet end to your baby's meal, try strained fruit or small pieces of fruit and plain yogurt instead of a sugary dessert.

Honey, Not Now!

Honey is not a better choice than sugar. Babies under 12 months old should never be fed honey. That's because honey may contain dangerous spores of bacteria called *Clostridium botulinum*, which can grow in the baby's intestinal tract and potentially cause life-threatening infant botulism. A baby's intestinal tract is unable to destroy these harmful bacteria, but an older child's intestinal tract is able to prevent the growth of these spores and their toxin. For safety reasons and because you're shaping your baby's taste preferences, don't give your baby honey or products made with honey, such as honey graham crackers.

What Should My Baby Eat Each Day?

By 9 to 12 months old, your baby should have a regular meal pattern that includes breast milk or iron-fortified infant formula and many different nutritious foods. A day's eating should consist of three small meals plus snacks, with daily servings from each of the food groups.

The daily amounts shown below will help your baby get the nutrients she needs. Amounts are approximate as babies' appetites vary. Look for signs that your baby has had enough, and stop feeding at that point. This will help prevent your baby from eating too much and gaining excessive weight.

Daily Eating Plan

Food Group	Foods	Daily Amounts
Dairy	Mainly breast milk or iron-fortified infant formula Also plain full-fat yogurt, cheese, cottage cheese (preferably no-salt-added)	Breast milk on demand; 3–4 formula feedings a day, with 4–6 ounces formula at each feeding
Grains	Iron-fortified infant cereal or hot cereal, low-sugar cold cereal (such as original Cheerios®), pasta, rice, small pieces of bread, crackers, teething biscuits	4–6 tablespoons* infant cereal a day A few bites or tablespoons of other grains a day, including whole-grain bread and cereal
Vegetables	Colorful and plain pureed, mashed or chopped cooked vegetables, such as sweet potatoes, carrots, tomatoes, zucchini, green beans, peas, spinach, broccoli	3–4 tablespoons a day
Fruits	Mashed or chopped fruit such as banana, melon, papaya, peach, blueberries, strawberries, quartered grapes	3–4 tablespoons a day
Protein Foods	Strained or finely chopped cooked lean meat, chicken, turkey, fish, egg yolk, tofu, mashed beans	1–3 tablespoons a day

* 1 tablespoon equals 3 teaspoons. A tablespoon is about the size of a woman's thumb.

What's the Right Portion Size?

Each baby's appetite is different so there really is no "correct" portion size. But very few parents underfeed their babies. Here again, the baby will give you a sign. Just provide enough food until she turns away. Never coax or force feed. The meal should be over when your baby's no longer interested in eating, not when you think she's had enough.

Like Parent, Like Child—Eat Your Fruits and Veggies

By the time a baby reaches 1 year old, she has likely been fed lots of pureed or strained fruits and vegetables. Eating these types of foods is a good practice for preventing childhood obesity. But as a baby starts to eat more regular table foods, she may be offered fewer servings of fruits and vegetables because of the way the rest of the family eats. Eating less of these foods is not healthy for the baby or the family.

Contrary to popular belief, children who are offered a variety of fruits and vegetables enjoy eating them. But your own attitude counts. Studies show that children are influenced by their parents' eating habits and are more likely to eat the same foods that their mom and dad eat. That's why it's so important to set a good example for your family. Let them see you eating good-for-you foods. If you enjoy fruits and vegetables, they may too! It may not happen overnight, but in time you'll see the change.

What About Fat?

Although adults may limit high-fat foods to help prevent weight gain, a baby's diet should not be restricted in fat. A baby needs fat for proper growth and brain development during the first year of life. Fat is an important source of energy, or calories, that a baby needs to keep up with her rapid growth. Fat also allows her brain to increase in size. Nerves in the baby's brain and body are lengthening and connecting with each other—a complex process that requires fat.

Although whole cow's milk contains fat, it should not be given to a baby until after age 1. That's because cow's milk is low in iron, too high in sodium for a baby's needs, and has too much protein for her to digest properly. Breast milk and formula contain enough of the healthy fats and other nutrients she needs.

When your baby reaches 6 months old, complement the breast milk or formula with a variety of solid foods. Nutritious choices that also provide some fat include strained or finely chopped meat, egg yolk, full-fat yogurt and cheese. Be sure to introduce foods one at a time, with three to five days between each new food. See "Getting Started on Solid Foods" on page 55.

Babies need fat for proper growth and brain development.

Expect a Food Rebellion, but Don't Fight Back

At 9 to 12 months old, many babies suddenly rebel against eating. Since growth slows during this time, the body requires less food. So if your baby has less of an appetite at this age, that's OK.

Don't force your baby to eat. Allow her to eat as much or as little as she wants instead of as much as you think she needs. If she refuses to eat, she just isn't hungry. She won't starve if she skips a meal.

Ellyn Satter, an authority on child feeding and eating, explains feeding as a division of responsibility: Your role is to provide your baby with wholesome, nutritious foods. Your baby's role is to decide how much to eat.

When your baby is beyond 6 months, you may find that she starts rejecting new foods. Scientists call this food neophobia—a fear of, or reluctance to try, new foods. It continues into the toddler and preschool years and starts to decrease with age.

How a parent responds to the challenge of food neophobia can influence which tastes a child comes to find acceptable. Offer a new food without comment, and see if she will taste it. If she refuses it, or spits it out, don't get upset. It may take 10 to 15 exposures to a new food before your child accepts it. Be prepared to try the food again at another meal.

Studies show that parental food choices can influence your baby's acceptance of wholesome foods. If you offer your baby a new food, it may help if you eat a bite or two of the same food in front of her, so she knows it's a food you like. Since she's watching and learning from what you do, this is a great opportunity to be a role model on eating healthful foods.

Mealtime Pleasure, Not Pressure

It's not a good idea to reward eating with praise or show disapproval when your baby doesn't finish her meal. Early on, a baby begins to recognize her parents' intense interest in what and how much she eats. The baby starts to realize that eating all the food on her plate brings approval. "What a good girl, you finished your whole dinner!" Mom or dad jumps for joy when the baby eats, but is upset and unhappy when the baby refuses to eat.

It's inappropriate for a baby to eat to please her parent or caregiver. What's appropriate is for a baby to eat because she's hungry and to stop eating when she's had enough. A baby brought up with this concept in mind will be much less likely to gain excess weight.

Make Meals a Family Affair

At about 9 months, your baby's likely starting to eat finely chopped foods or small pieces of soft foods. She's not yet ready to eat everything the rest of the family eats, but she can certainly join you at the table during family meals.

At this age, your baby may be trying to feed herself with a spoon. Encourage her to do so, even though it will be messy at first. Give her finger foods that she can eat with her hands. See "Finger Foods for Babies" on page 57.

Eating family meals together on most, if not all, days of the week can help children stay at a healthy weight. Be sure to include your baby, even if she isn't quite able to feed herself completely. Making family meals a habit is a wise investment in preventing childhood obesity.

If cooking isn't your strong point, try not to rely on fast-food and take-out meals for your family. Meals prepared outside the home are often higher in calories and have a larger portion size than similar meals cooked at home. Frequently eating fast-food meals can increase the risk of childhood obesity.

Instead of eating out or bringing take-out foods home, search the Internet for simple and healthful home-cooked recipes your family will enjoy. You'll find some recipes in the *Chef's Select Cookbook* on the Shape Up America!® website at *www.shapeup.org*.

CHAPTER 5

Rapid Weight Gain—A Risk Factor for Childhood Obesity

Hold the Reins on Rapid Weight Gain

Babies gain weight as part of their normal growth, and they do it at an amazing rate. They typically double their birth weight by about 5 months old, and triple their birth weight by 12 months. But babies who gain weight too rapidly may be at risk of becoming obese as a child.

According to a Harvard study, babies who gain weight too quickly in their first six months have a greater chance of becoming obese by age 3. Babies born to mothers with any type of diabetes have an increased risk of childhood obesity, so their weight should be monitored every couple of months. A German study on babies of mothers with type 1 (insulin-dependent) diabetes or gestational (pregnancy-related) diabetes found that babies who gained weight too rapidly during the first four months of life had six times the risk of becoming obese later on.

The tables below show the range of weight and length that's considered "normal" for infants up to 12 months old. They're based on percentiles, a measurement that allows a pediatrician to compare your baby to many other babies of the same age and sex.

A normal weight ranges from the 5th percentile—the low end of the range—up to the 95th percentile—the high end of the range. For example, if a baby is at the

90th percentile for weight, this means that he weighs more than 90 percent of babies of the same age and sex.

Similarly, a normal length ranges from the 5th percentile up to the 95th percentile compared to babies of the same age and sex. For example, if a baby is at the 90th percentile for length, this means that he's longer than 90 percent of all babies of the same age and sex. Length is measured instead of height since babies are measured lying down, facing up.

There are separate weight and length values for boys and girls since they grow at different rates. To use the tables below, find the age in months of your baby girl or boy, and read across that line for the expected range of weight-for-age and length-for-age.

For all babies, 90 percent will fall within the normal range for weight and length. If your baby falls outside this range, it's important to visit a pediatrician for further evaluation. The doctor can assess if a baby whose growth is below the 5th percentile is experiencing "failure to thrive," and if a baby whose weight is above the 95th percentile is developing obesity.

Girls' Normal Weight and Length

Age	Weight (pounds)		Length (inches)	
	Low	High	Low	High
Birth	5.6	8.9	18.1	20.6
1 month	7.3	11.5	19.9	22.4
2 months	9.1	13.9	21.1	23.8
3 months	10.4	15.8	22.2	24.9
4 months	11.5	17.3	23.0	25.8
5 months	12.4	18.6	23.8	26.6
6 months	13.2	19.7	24.4	27.3
7 months	13.8	20.6	25.0	28.0
8 months	14.3	21.4	25.5	28.6
9 months	14.9	22.2	26.1	29.2
10 months	15.3	22.9	26.5	29.7
11 months	15.7	23.6	27.0	30.3
12 months	16.2	24.2	27.5	30.8

Figures are derived from the CDC/WHO data tables used in weight-for-age and length-for-age growth charts for girls.

Boys' Normal Weight and Length

Age	Weight (pounds)		Length (inches)	
	Low	High	Low	High
Birth	5.7	9.3	18.4	20.9
1 month	7.8	12.2	20.3	22.8
2 months	9.9	15.0	21.7	24.3
3 months	11.5	17.0	22.9	25.5
4 months	12.8	18.5	23.8	26.5
5 months	13.7	19.8	24.6	27.3
6 months	14.5	20.9	25.2	28.0
7 months	15.2	21.8	25.8	28.6
8 months	15.8	22.6	26.4	29.2
9 months	16.3	23.4	26.9	29.8
10 months	16.8	24.1	27.4	30.3
11 months	17.3	24.7	27.8	30.9
12 months	17.7	25.4	28.3	31.4

Figures are derived from the CDC/WHO data tables used in weight-for-age and length-for-age growth charts for boys.

What Causes Rapid Weight Gain?

Rapid weight gain could be due to your baby's daily diet, amount of exercise and sleep routine. Or there could be a medical explanation. To help you figure out what might be causing excess weight gain, make an appointment to see your baby's pediatrician. Prepare for the visit by answering these questions:

- Did you introduce solid foods before your child was 6 months old?

- Do you give your baby juice or sugary drinks regularly?

- Do you feed your baby on a set schedule rather than feeding him on demand or only when he's hungry?

- Is your baby inactive most of the time?

- Does your baby get less than 12 hours of sleep a day?

- Do you engage in less than one hour of daily active play with your child?

If you answered "yes" to any of these questions, your baby may be on his way to becoming overweight or obese. Speak with your pediatrician or healthcare provider about ways to slow your child's rate of weight gain. Here are some tips to help you get started:

- If your baby has started eating solid foods, discuss your baby's diet to make sure he's consuming the right amounts and types of foods and drinks. A national study of children under age 4 found that inappropriate foods such as French fries, presweetened cereals, and sugary and caffeinated soda are often fed to babies as young as 3 months old.

- Avoid giving your baby juice, fruit drinks or sugary soda. Fruit is nutritious and more satisfying than juice.

- Tune in to your baby's signs that he's hungry, such as opening his mouth or leaning forward, and stop feeding him when he shows signs that he's full, such as turning away and losing interest in eating. If you bottle feed, try feeding your baby a little less at each meal. To start, offer 6 ounces of formula instead of 8 ounces. Feed him more only if he signals that he's still hungry.

- Don't cut calories by adding water to the formula, unless advised how best to do so by your baby's pediatrician or healthcare provider. Diluting formula with water could deprive your baby of important nutrients needed for proper growth and development.

- Feed your baby foods prepared at home. Eating out often and feeding your baby restaurant foods, especially fast foods and drinks, may contribute to rapid weight gain.

- Make sure your baby gets at least 12 hours of sleep in 24 hours. For more information on sleep, see "Lack of Sleep—A Link to Childhood Obesity" on page 73.

- Increase physical activity to burn up calories. Babies need to be active. For ideas on how to help your child become more physically active, see "The Benefits of Physical Activity Start Early in Life" on page 79.

Growth Rate Matters–Keep It Steady

Some people think a big baby is a healthy baby. It's true that a certain amount of fat is needed for your baby's growth and development, but babies with too much fat have a greater chance of becoming obese later in life.

Yet, healthy babies come in all shapes and sizes. What matters more than size is steady growth. To help you know if your baby's growth is progressing at a healthy rate, it's important that your baby's doctor, or healthcare provider, weigh and measure your baby every couple of months.

The AAP recommends that your doctor use standardized charts to record your baby's growth in four areas: head circumference, length, weight and weight-for-length. The growth chart that most informs the risk of childhood obesity is the weight-for-length chart. The doctor weighs your baby, measures the baby's length and plots the measurements on percentile lines on the chart. The percentiles show how your baby's growing compared to babies of the same age and sex. Ideally, a baby's growth pattern, or the rate that he gains weight and grows in length, should be proportional to each other. That means the percentile line on the weight-for-length chart should stay about the same over time.

For example, a 9-month-old boy weighs 24.8 pounds and is 30.1 inches in length. His weight-for-length measurements put him at the 95th percentile, which means he is heavier than 95 percent of other boys his age. However, it's important to know the baby's growth history. If his rate of growth was steady over time, around the 95th percentile, it's possible he weighs as much as he does simply because he's a bigger baby. But if his weight-for-length measurements were at the 50th percentile most of his life and have now jumped up to the 95th percentile, that's a cause for concern.

If his measurements stayed within the normal range but jumped up from his usual 50th percentile to the 75th percentile, it should also be checked by the baby's pediatrician.

A rapid increase may signal the onset of obesity, whether it's within or above the normal weight range.

A visit to the pediatrician every two months will allow the doctor to monitor your baby's growth rate over time.

A steady growth pattern is usually OK, even in a big baby. Big jumps in growth rate may be a sign of obesity.

CHAPTER 6

Lack of Sleep–A Link to Childhood Obesity

Sleep is Divine

For many Americans, getting enough shut-eye seems to be a welcome prospect but an unlikely reality. Sleep studies have shown that over the past 20+ years, teens, children and babies have been getting less sleep, mainly due to later bedtimes. Increasing evidence on infants and young children has linked shorter sleep time with a greater risk of childhood obesity. Infants should get 12 or more hours of sleep in 24 hours to protect against childhood obesity.

At 2:00 a.m., the mom of 3-month-old Samantha called. "Dr. Eden, my baby just woke up. My mother told me that if I added cereal to my daughter's bottle in the evening, she would sleep through the night. What do you think?"

I answered, "No studies have ever shown that feeding a baby cereal in a bottle will help her sleep through the night. Your baby's ability to sleep is more due to her age than what she eats. Be patient. In a couple of months, she should be able to sleep longer at night."

It's unrealistic to expect a 3- or 4-month-old baby to sleep through the night. Yet, in one study, half of the moms surveyed believed that feeding their babies solid foods would make them sleep longer. This belief is often passed down through the generations, but it's not supported by science.

In fact, feeding solid foods too early, including adding infant cereal to a bottle, may be harmful. It increases the chance of your baby choking since she may not yet have the ability to swallow foods while lying down. Plus, the digestive tract of a baby who's only a few months old may not be developed enough to process solid foods. Feeding her solids could make her feel ill, get diarrhea or vomit. It could also cause your baby to consume too little nutritious breast milk or formula. Introducing solids too early can lead to overfeeding, which puts your baby at greater risk of childhood obesity.

Soothing Strategies for a Better Sleep

If your baby's not sleeping well, in rare cases there may be a medical cause that will need the attention of your pediatrician. For otherwise healthy babies, here are some strategies that can help you soothe your baby and improve her sleep:

Day Light, Dark Night

- Exposing your baby to sunlight in the morning and afternoon can help set her internal clock so it synchronizes with the day–night cycle. This will help her sleep at bedtime and stay asleep longer.

- To help your baby sleep at night, make sure her room is completely dark.

Soothing Bedtime Rituals

- Some cultures use massage to soothe babies and get them ready for sleep. One study showed that babies who received 14 days of massage therapy starting at 2 weeks old had more mature sleep patterns and higher levels of the nighttime sleep hormone, melatonin, at 12 weeks old. Consider massaging your baby to help her get to sleep.

- If your baby finds a bath soothing, and not stimulating, include a warm bath as part of your bedtime calming routine.

- In the U.S. and western societies, the ideal is for babies to learn how to fall asleep on their own. To achieve this, don't let your baby fall asleep in your arms. At bedtime, put her in her bed before she has fallen asleep. Note that some cultures expect the parent to soothe a baby to sleep. Some parents may want to decide whether to soothe their baby or let their baby soothe herself to sleep. You can also discuss sleep issues with your baby's pediatrician.

Day and Night Routines

- A regular sleeping schedule and bedtime routine can help lull your baby to sleep. If bedtime is too early, your baby may not be tired enough to go to sleep. If bedtime is too late, she may seem energetic but is actually overtired. If your baby's bedtime varies and she's not sleeping well, try to switch to a consistent bedtime. Establish a soothing bedtime ritual to help her wind down. For example, read a story, sing a lullaby, then give your baby a kiss goodnight.

- Lengthen the time between your baby's last nap of the day and her bedtime to help her fall asleep more easily.

- Younger or smaller infants need to eat during the night, so that's to be expected. If your infant is over 6 months old and growing well, but is still waking up at night wanting to feed, give your baby her last meal of the day at a later time. Try feeding her between 10:00 p.m. and midnight and see if that helps her sleep longer during the night.

- If your baby still wakes up too soon after her final feeding, delay feeding her again by using tactics that lengthen the time between feedings, such as changing her diaper or rocking her quietly in a rocking chair. Studies show that this approach can help babies sleep quietly from midnight to 5:00 a.m., although it may take several weeks for this delaying method to succeed.

- Follow a daily, age-appropriate physical activity routine to help your baby sleep better at night. See "The Benefits of Physical Activity Start Early in Life" on page 79.

Nighttime Agreement

- If there are two parents who might help out when your baby wakes up at night, be sure to agree on the tactics you will both use to soothe your baby and put her back to sleep.

- First make sure your baby's awake. Your baby may make noises or even call out while sleeping. Avoid disturbing her until you're absolutely sure she's awake and needs attention.

- Keep things calm, not animated, to encourage her to go back to sleep as soon as possible. Talk softly or sing. If you pick her up to rock her that's fine, but don't bounce her or start playing a game.

- Be consistent in your approach. Make sure everyone who takes care of the baby agrees on how to get her back to sleep, so she's not confused.

- Think about your comfort level with the crying-it-out approach. For sleep-deprived parents, allowing your baby to cry herself to sleep may seem appealing. But many parents are not comfortable doing this. This approach is meant to help the baby learn to go to sleep on her own. It's done in steps and doesn't mean letting your baby cry all night without giving her any attention. In our opinion, crying it out is not appropriate for babies under 6 months old or for small babies, and is considered controversial in older infants. If you want to try it, speak with your baby's pediatrician first to see if it's appropriate for her.

A Note About Crying

Crying is a form of exercise in an infant and may signal that your baby's not getting enough physical activity during the day. Since exposure to sunlight is beneficial for nighttime sleep, exercising your baby outdoors during the day may be especially helpful in getting her to sleep through the night.

Sometimes crying can really get on adults' nerves. Shaken baby syndrome happens when a frustrated parent or caregiver loses control and violently shakes a crying baby. Shaking a baby is very dangerous and can cause blindness, seizures, brain damage or death. Make sure that anyone responsible for your baby's care is warned not to shake your baby.

TV, Sleep and Childhood Obesity

What does screen time, which includes TV, computers, DVDs, cell phones, tablets and video games have to do with preventing obesity in an infant? A lot. The more hours a baby sits in front of the TV and other screens, the higher the risk of obesity.

One recent survey showed that by 1 year old, half of all infants were watching at least one hour of TV each day. The AAP recommends no TV for children under 2 years old: "An infant's brain develops rapidly and learns best by interacting with people, not screens."

Many parents find that sitting their baby in a high chair in front of a TV, often with a snack, allows them time to do necessary chores. We understand, but it's better to find an alternative to TV. How about asking an older brother or sister or family member to play with her or read her a book? Or better yet, choose a safe area for your baby to crawl or walk around so she can safely explore her surroundings while you do your chores. This will burn up calories and keep her more active, reducing her chances of gaining weight too rapidly.

Watching TV may lead to obesity by encouraging inactivity and undermining sleep. A baby needs a total of 12 or more hours of sleep a day. Noise, light and distractions, such as a TV, can affect how well and how long the baby sleeps. When it's your baby's naptime or bedtime, the bedroom needs to be quiet and dark. If your baby shares a bedroom, it's best not to have a TV in the room. Or at least turn the TV off when it's time for your baby to sleep.

CHAPTER 7

The Benefits of Physical Activity Start Early in Life

Babies Need Exercise

Physical activity is important for a baby's health and motor skill development. Although research on physical activity in babies is limited, a 2008 report by the Institute of Medicine (IOM) suggests that physical activity during infancy may help control excessive weight gain. Daily physical activity promotes gross motor development—the ability to use large muscle groups, such as those in the arms and legs—to move the body. But according to the IOM report, obese babies may be delayed in reaching gross motor milestones, and as a result, may be less physically active later in childhood. For other babies, low levels of physical activity can lead to obesity.

The report recommends that babies get sufficient time each day to move around and explore their surroundings indoors and outdoors, under adult supervision. Movements such as reaching, crawling and learning to walk are some of the main ways that your baby can use up energy (burn calories).

You can help your baby be active by providing space for him to move, playing with him on the floor and encouraging him to move around and explore. These movements burn calories and can help him maintain a healthy weight.

There are a number of developmental milestones your baby needs to reach to help him grow strong and gain the skills to be physically active. Here is what to look for at each stage during infancy.

Note that these milestones are based on average ranges of growth and development. Your baby may reach these milestones sooner or later than the ages shown here. If you're concerned your baby may be experiencing a true delay in development, contact his pediatrician.

Physical Activity Developmental Milestones

Age	What to Look For
Newborn	Movement is not controlled. Your baby's head is flopped to one side or the other when he's on his back. It's difficult for him to turn his head from one side to the other when lying on his tummy. He can stand briefly on his legs while held upright.
1 month	When wide awake and lying on his tummy, your baby will try to hold his head up. When on his back and pulled up to sitting, his head will lag (chin won't tuck in toward his chest). Your baby can stand longer on his legs when held upright, and he may make a stepping movement.
1–2 months	Your baby will start to swipe and reach at things placed in front of him. He'll be able to lift his head, and possibly his chest, off the floor when placed on his tummy. He'll be able to hold his head in the center when lying on his back.
2–3 months	Your baby starts to reach for toys. His head is centered with chin tucked when lying on his back. He can hold his head up and prop himself up on his forearms when placed on his tummy. He's able to stand with straight legs when held upright, with your hands around his chest.

Age	What to Look For
3–4 months	Your baby may roll from his stomach to his back. He may start to sit up with propping and support. He reaches with his hands more purposefully and swipes at nearby objects. He'll start to hold his head up fairly steadily. While lying on his back, he'll lift his head up with chin tucked and can bring his knees up to his hands. Your baby may start to stand while you hold his hands rather than his chest.
4–5 months	Lying on his back, your baby lifts his head and shoulders. He rolls from stomach to back. He sits with head and back steady with support. He enjoys being pulled up to standing position. Your baby is able to hold his bottle or other objects with both hands or one hand. He begins to transfer objects from one hand to the other. He starts to reach for and grasp objects.
5–6 months	Lying on his back, your baby can grab his feet. He can roll from his back to his stomach. He sits without much support. He holds a toy well. He reaches and swipes with one arm at a time. Your baby begins to manipulate objects in his hands. He may grasp small objects off a flat surface. On his stomach, he starts to creep forward or backward with his legs and steers with his arms. If you use a playpen, stock it with interesting, safe objects such as rattles, balls and plastic toys.
6–7 months	Your baby sits well with little support. He can grasp with his thumb and fingers. He creeps and then starts to crawl. He rolls over from back to stomach and stomach to back. He stands with support and gets himself up into a sitting position. He holds and handles a spoon or cup.
7–8 months	Your baby sits without support. He crawls forward and backward. He stands well with support. He pulls himself up to a standing position using furniture to help. Once standing, he usually can't get back down on his own.
8–9 months	Your baby has mastered a pincer grasp with his thumb and forefinger. He crawls efficiently, even when holding a toy. He cruises along furniture and can crawl upstairs. He may stand alone for a moment. He can pull himself up to standing, often in the middle of the night, and calls for help to get back down.

Age	What to Look For
9–10 months	Your baby stands with little or no support. He walks a few steps holding on and cruises along holding onto furniture. He climbs up and down from a low chair. He can now sit down from a standing position. He can carry objects in one hand.
10–11 months	Your baby stands alone. He begins to climb stairs. He walks with only a little support, holding one of your hands. He begins to pull his socks off. He's able to use a spoon to feed himself and splatter the walls.
11–12 months	Your baby walks alone for a few steps. He climbs up and down stairs and may climb out of his playpen or crib. He helps undress himself. He likes to crawl rapidly around the house. He goes from standing to sitting easily and speedily.

Source: Adapted from Eden AN. Positive Parenting: Raising Healthy Children from Birth to Three Years. New York: Hatherleigh Press; 2007.

Let's Play!

Not all babies are naturally active. Many are sedentary and must be encouraged to exercise. The earlier you start your baby exercising, the better. In fact, as soon as you get home from the hospital, you can help your baby begin to develop strength, agility and good muscle tone. One precaution is to make sure you support your baby's head during the first month or two because it's still quite wobbly.

Try these suggested exercises for babies up to 12 months old.

0 to 3 Months

Tummy time is important when your baby's awake since this can help him develop strong muscles. Place your baby on his tummy several times each day so he can practice lifting his head, eventually holding it up. However, when you put your baby to sleep, it's safest if you put him on his back.

Your baby will enjoy being handled and bounced up and down on your lap. The earlier you start, the stronger and more agile he will become. To strengthen muscles in your baby's legs, place him on his back and pump his legs gently as if he's riding a bicycle. To strengthen his large, central core muscles, carry him around in various positions, not just up on your shoulder. Infant carriers or slings can be used for this purpose. Alternate having your baby face forward or backward in his sling as this will exercise different muscles.

Consider hanging a colorful crib device over your baby's crib. Sturdy devices, such as cradle gyms, have rings and bells attached that will encourage your baby to reach for objects. This will allow him to exercise his arms. As your baby becomes more skilled at hitting or grasping the cradle gym toys, reinforce his accomplishments with a cheer or a hug.

To see a video of the following songs and games you can play with your 0- to 3-month-old baby, visit the Shape Up America!® website at *www.shapeup.org* and select "exercise videos" from the Resources menu.

The first game is *Tap Tap, Rub Rub Rub*. The lyrics are simple, but this little game will encourage stretching and across-the-body communication that involves the right and left brain. With your baby lying on his back, start by holding the soles of his feet together, tapping them twice against each other and then rubbing them against each other as you rhythmically say *Tap Tap, Rub Rub Rub*. Repeat. Alternate criss-crossing the feet as you slowly say, *Criss Cross, Criss Cross*. Then uncross the legs and gently stretch out the baby's legs as you slowly say *Strrrrrretch*.

Now repeat the whole process with the baby's arms. Then choose one hand and the opposite foot to repeat the process. Choose the other hand and opposite foot to repeat the process a final time.

> *Tap Tap, Rub Rub Rub.*
> *Tap Tap, Rub Rub Rub.*
> *Criss Cross, Criss Cross.*
> *Strrrrrretch!*

The next game is *A-Bouncing We Will Go*. Hold your baby securely on your lap and act out the song's lyrics, first gently bouncing the baby, then rocking the baby and then tickling the baby, as you say or sing the words.

> *A-bouncing we will go, a-bouncing we will go,*
> *High-ho the dairy oh, a-bouncing we will go.*
>
> *A-rocking we will go, a-rocking we will go,*
> *High-ho the dairy oh, a-rocking we will go.*
>
> *A-tickling we will go, a-tickling we will go,*
> *High-ho the dairy oh, a-tickling we will go.*

The last game for this very young age group is *X Marks the Spot*. For a newborn and very young baby, tummy time is especially important. For this game you can place your baby on his tummy. As you touch his back in various places, your baby will feel your touches and respond. This will give him a chance to exercise his neck and back muscles as you say the words:

> *X marks the spot, (With your finger, draw a large "X" on baby's back.)*
> *With a dot and a dot, (Draw dots on baby's back.)*
> *And a dash and a dash, (Draw dashes on baby's back.)*
> *And a big question mark. (Draw a question mark on baby's back.)*

Up and down, (Draw a zigzag up and down baby's back.)

Round and round. (Draw circles on baby's back.)

Crack an egg on your head, (Place your hands on baby's head.)

Let the yolk run down.

(Run your hands down baby's body from head to toe.)

Crack an egg on your head, (Place your hands on baby's head.)

Let the yolk run down.

(Run your hands down baby's body from head to toe.)

3 to 6 Months

Babies who are 3 to 6 months old love to exercise. Encouraging your baby to explore and exercise will prevent him from becoming sedentary. At this age your baby's muscles are increasing in strength, coordination is building, and brain development is continuing at a rapid pace. Exercising and interacting with your baby support these beneficial changes.

Encourage your baby to use all of his muscles by exposing him to a variety of exercises each day. Here are some ways to do this:

- **Crib devices:** Place your baby on his back. Hang a cradle gym or toys, such as a mirror and rattle, in front of him so he can reach for and grasp these objects. This is a useful form of physical activity.

- **Turn-over games:** Babies never seem to get tired of turning over again and again, so this activity can be lots of fun for your baby. It's a wonderful form of exercise because it strengthens your baby's muscles and increases his agility or ability to change positions.

- **Kicking toys:** Attach large cuddly kicking toys to the inside of the crib. Your baby will enjoy kicking at the toys and grabbing for them. This will help him develop strength in his legs and will keep him happy and busy.

- **Standing:** When babies reach 3 to 6 months, most can support their own weight when standing, while they're held up to steady them. Carefully place your baby on his feet each day to help him develop his leg strength and improve his large-muscle coordination. There's no truth to the tale that standing a baby up early will cause bowlegs.

- **Creeping and rocking:** When babies reach 5 to 6 months, they start to creep or push themselves along forward or backward. Several times a day, put your baby on the floor or in a playpen so he has space to practice these new skills.

To see a video of the following songs and games you can play with your 3- to 6-month-old baby, visit the Shape Up America!® website at *www.shapeup.org* and select "exercise videos" from the Resources menu.

The first game is *Patty Cake*. It encourages interaction, touching and a wide range of motions. Start by taking your baby's hands in your own and clapping them together as you say the words:

> *Patty cake, patty cake, baker's man.*
> *Bake me a cake as fast as you can.*
> *Roll it, (Make a rolling motion with baby's arms or legs.)*
> *And pat it, (Pat your baby's tummy.)*
> *And mark it with a "B," (Write a "B" on baby's tummy.)*
> *And put it in the oven for baby and me!*

You can modify *Patty Cake* by using your baby's first initial and his own name in the last line. As your baby grows older, you can vary the motions.

The next game is *Tick Tock, Tick Tock, I'm a Little Cuckoo Clock*. Your baby will enjoy being rocked and then lifted up into the air as the clock cuckoos. This game will help your baby eventually learn to count. If you have other kids, they might like to "cuckoo" along with you.

Tick tock, tick tock, I'm a little cuckoo clock, (Rock baby back and forth.)
Tick tock, tick tock, now we're striking one o'clock.
Cuckoo! (Lift baby into the air once to mark the time.)

Tick tock, tick tock, I'm a little cuckoo clock,
Tick tock, tick tock, now we're striking two o'clock.
Cuckoo! Cuckoo! (Lift baby into the air twice to mark the time.)

If your baby's having fun, continue the game until you reach twelve o'clock.

The last game for this age group is *What Shall We Do With a Tiny Baby?*

What shall we do with a tiny baby?
What shall we do with a tiny baby?
What shall we do with a tiny baby?
Early in the morning.

Roll him around and tickle him all over, (Roll and tickle baby.)
Roll him around and tickle him all over,
Roll him around and tickle him all over,
Early in the morning.

Heave ho! And up he rises, (Lift baby up.)
Heave ho! And up he rises,
Heave ho! And up he rises,
Early in the morning.

6 to 9 Months

What your baby needs at this age is the space to move around—to creep, crawl, swing around and cruise. The most important thing you can provide is a clean and safe space for him to explore. That may mean blocking electrical outlets, removing items from tables that he might be able to pull down such as lamps with cords, and dangerous objects he might put in his mouth.

A 6- to 9-month-old enjoys being physically handled. He loves to be swung in the air, bounced up and down, and is very happy when you get on the floor to play with him, crawl around and chase him. By promoting and encouraging daily physical activity at this early age and beyond, you will improve your baby's health and help prevent the development of obesity.

At this stage, babies love many types of games: rhythm games, dropping games, cause-and-effect games such as turning a light on and off, floor games, hide-and-seek games, and building and stacking games. We recommend letting your baby play in bare feet instead of shoes when indoors since it can help him feel the ground better.

Some babies at this age are already above a healthy weight. An obese 6- to 9-month-old is content to sit or lie around, possibly drinking a bottle of milk or juice to keep him occupied. A vicious cycle now begins: The fatter the baby, the less active he becomes. The less active he is, the fewer calories he burns, which may lead him to become even heavier. It requires extra effort to encourage an inactive, heavy baby to exercise in order to break this vicious cycle.

To see a video of the following songs and games you can play with your 6- to 9-month-old baby, visit the Shape Up America!® website at *www.shapeup.org* and select "exercise videos" from the Resources menu.

The first is *Bumpin' Up and Down in My Little Red Wagon*, a game that has a snappy tempo. Start with your baby in your lap, facing you, with your hands holding him securely around his waist.

> *Bumpin' up and down in my little red wagon,*
> *(Bounce your baby in time to the tune.)*
> *Bumpin' up and down in my little red wagon,*
> *Bumpin' up and down in my little red wagon,*
> *Won't you be my darlin'?*

> *One wheel's off and the axle's broken, (Lean baby side to side.)*
> *One wheel's off and the axle's broken,*
> *One wheel's off and the axle's broken,*
> *Won't you be my darlin'?*

You can also stand and march around holding your baby as you sing this tune. As he gets older and can stand with support or stand alone, you can march together and act out the song.

The next game is called *The Grand Old Duke of York*. You can hold your baby and go up and down yourself, sit your baby on your lap and move his arms up and down, or, when he's older, have him eventually stand to reach up and down and act out the song.

> *The Grand Old Duke of York, (March in place.)*
> *He had ten thousand men.*
> *He marched them up to the top of the hill,*
> *(Lift baby up or reach arms up high.)*
> *And he marched them down again. (Lower baby or arms.)*

> *'Cause when you're up, you're up, (Lift baby up or reach arms up high.)*
> *And when you're down, you're down. (Lower baby or arms.)*

And when you're only half way up, (Hold arms or child at waist height.)
You're neither up nor down. (Reach and lift up and down again.)

For the final game, *If You're Happy and You Know It*, start with the words and motions shown here, and then move on to ideas of your own. As your child grows older, encourage him to make up his own motions.

If you're happy and you know it, stretch up high, (Reach up to the sky.)
If you're happy and you know it, stretch up high,
If you're happy and you know it, and you really want to show it,
If you're happy and you know it, stretch up high.

If you're happy and you know it, stretch down low,
        (Reach down to the floor.)
If you're happy and you know it, stretch down low,
If you're happy and you know it, and you really want to show it,
If you're happy and you know it, stretch down low.

If you're happy and you know it, shout "Hooray!"
If you're happy and you know it, shout "Hooray!"
If you're happy and you know it, and you really want to show it,
If you're happy and you know it, shout "Hooray!"

You can add almost any action at the end of the phrase, *If you're happy and you know it.* For example you can give him a shaker or a rattle and sing, *If you're happy and you know it, shake up high.* Or you can add *clap your hands* or *stamp your feet.*

9 to 12 Months

A 9- to 12-month-old begins to stand without support, walks with and sometimes without support, climbs up and down the stairs, and can easily go from standing to sitting. He's able to pick up and handle small objects. At this age, a baby needs the space and opportunity to use his muscles to build strength and develop coordination, balance and agility, which is the ability to change direction.

Take your baby outdoors as often as possible. The goal for outdoor activity is to carry your baby around less, take fewer trips with your baby in a carriage or stroller, and let him walk and play more. Roughhouse activities such as tumbling will strengthen his muscles and help him become more active and agile. When outdoors, it's OK to expose your baby's skin to sunlight for about 15 minutes. This will boost his vitamin D levels, which is essential for building strong bones. But if your baby's outdoors for longer than 15 minutes, apply sun protection lotion liberally to his skin.

For indoor activity, be sure to child-proof your home. Most accidents can be prevented by removing objects that might be dangerous. Your baby will love playing with a ball, but make sure it's large enough so he can't swallow it or choke on it. He might enjoy a football because it bounces around in every direction. Besides chasing the ball, your baby will start learning to throw and catch it.

When your baby is 9 to 12 months old, it's a good time to reassess the pattern of his growth. Visit your baby's pediatrician to have his growth checked. See "Growth Rate Matters—Keep It Steady" on page 70. If your baby's overweight, you can help slow down his weight gain by increasing his physical activity, especially outdoors.

One factor that can contribute to an inactive child is overprotection and excessive worry about his well-being. Discouraging physical activity due to fear of an accident can inadvertently damage a baby's natural curiosity and heighten the risk of childhood obesity, if it's not already present.

To see a video of the following songs and games you can play with your 9- to 12-month-old baby, visit the Shape Up America!® website at *www.shapeup.org* and select "exercise videos" from the Resources menu.

The first is *Open and Shut Them*, a game that teaches simple motions, body parts and concepts.

> *Open and shut them, open and shut them,*
> *Give a little clap, clap, clap.*
>
> *Open and shut them, open and shut them,*
> *Put them in your lap, lap, lap.*
>
> *Creep them, crawl them,*
> *Creep them, crawl them,*
> *Right up to your chin, chin, chin.*
>
> *Open up your little mouth,*
> *But do not let them in.*

Another familiar tune is *Head, Shoulders, Knees and Toes*. This song is stimulating to your baby and will help him learn the names of a few parts of the body. Lay your baby down and touch the named parts of his body as you sing along. Then repeat the song and assist your baby's own hands to touch his own body parts as you sing the song. Older kids might want to sing along too.

> *Head, shoulders, knees and toes, knees and toes,*
> *Head, shoulders, knees and toes, knees and toes.*

Eyes and ears and mouth and nose,
Head, shoulders, knees and toes, knees and toes.

The final game for ages 9 to 12 months is *The Wheels on the Bus*. There are many variations and different motions that you can make up. To start, you can move your baby's arms along with the song, or you can make the motions for your baby and encourage him to imitate you. Imitation is a clear indication that your baby's learning to recognize and understand words.

The wheels on the bus go round and round,
Round and round,
Round and round.
The wheels on the bus go round and round,
All through the town!

The horn on the bus goes beep, beep, beep,
Beep, beep, beep,
Beep, beep, beep.
The horn on the bus goes beep, beep, beep,
All through the town!

The children on the bus go up and down,
Up and down,
Up and down.
The children on the bus go up and down,
All through the town!

The babies on the bus go wah-wah-wah,
Wah-wah-wah,
Wah-wah-wah.
The babies on the bus go wah-wah-wah,
All through the town!

The wipers on the bus go swish-swish-swish,
Swish-swish-swish,
Swish-swish-swish.
The wipers on the bus go swish-swish-swish,
All through the town!

Note that all of these songs and games can be adapted for younger and older babies. For younger babies you can make the games simpler and move your baby's body for him. As your baby grows older, he'll learn the words and motions and eventually should be able to make his own variations. This encourages him to exercise his mind and imagination, as well as his body. Continue to interact with your baby as much as possible each day.

Chapter 8

Losing Weight After Giving Birth

Protect Your Future Children from Obesity

As a proud parent, you're probably quite busy taking care of your baby. Perhaps you've thought about returning to your prepregnancy weight but aren't ready to deal with it now. Maybe you've considered expanding your family in the future so your baby has a brother or sister to play with.

Keep in mind that in the U.S., most pregnancies are unplanned. Parents—yes, both parents—who have BMIs above 25 increase the chances that their future child will be overweight or obese. The best way to reduce the risk of childhood obesity is for both parents to reach a healthy weight before the next pregnancy. One strategy that can help moms reach their prepregnancy weight is to breastfeed.

Breastfeeding Helps You Lose Weight

Milk production requires a lot of energy (calories). Breastfeeding makes your body burn calories from your own fat stores, which can help you lose weight. Your body uses about 500 calories a day to produce enough breast milk for a 6-week-old baby. This increases to about 800 calories a day for a 4-month-old baby.

If you're exclusively breastfeeding, the calories burned are higher than if you supplement breast milk with infant formula or other foods. The older and bigger your baby is, the more calories your body will burn to produce enough milk to feed her and help her grow.

When your baby's 4 to 6 months old, she'll be drinking close to one quart of breast milk a day. To produce this large amount of milk, a breastfeeding mom burns her own stores of body fat laid down during pregnancy. So at this point, a mom who is exclusively breastfeeding is getting leaner.

Yet, the scale may not show that you're losing weight. That's because your body shifts to retaining water that's needed to make breast milk. The weight of the increased water hides the fat loss that's occurring and this makes it seem like you're not losing that much weight on the scale. But you're actually losing body fat no matter what the scale says.

Once you start to wean your baby onto solid foods, milk production and the number of calories burned decreases. If you haven't already done so, this may be a good time to work toward achieving a healthy weight.

How to Get Back to Your Prepregnancy Weight

You don't have to wait until your baby's weaned to start losing weight. After about two months of breastfeeding, most women can take steps to actively lose weight, provided they do it slowly. A weight loss of about 1 to 1.5 pounds a week shouldn't affect your milk production. It's a good idea to first check with your doctor to make sure your milk production is adequate and your baby's growth is on track.

Keep in mind that fad diets that promise quick weight loss may not be nutritious and can make you produce less milk than your baby needs. Remember, too, that diets that omit fruits and vegetables are not beneficial to your baby's developing taste preferences. See "The Flavors of Breast Milk Shape Your Baby's Tastes" on page 28.

If you're formula feeding, give your body some time to recover from pregnancy. After about six weeks, consider slow and steady weight loss by eating healthfully, cutting down on portion sizes, and exercising. For example, put your baby in the stroller and take her for a walk. Whether you breastfeed or formula feed, it could take six months or longer to return to your prepregnancy weight.

Pregnancy may cause your body shape to change a bit, so be realistic with your goals and be kind to yourself.

For nutritious menu ideas and recipes, see Chapters 11–14 (starting on page 111).

CHAPTER 9

Special Topics for Parents

Postpartum Depression and Weight

Having a baby changes your life. Worries about being a new mom, lack of sleep, and social and hormonal changes lead many new moms to get teary-eyed and moody, and feel sad, anxious or overwhelmed. These are signs of the baby blues. These symptoms don't need treatment and should go away within a couple weeks. Try to get support to help with your baby's care and allow you to get some rest.

If the baby blues don't subside, and you feel extremely sad and worthless, lose your appetite, are unable to care for your baby, or even think about hurting your baby or yourself, you could be developing postpartum depression. Speak with your doctor or healthcare provider to find out if you're experiencing this potentially serious condition. Proper treatment, which may include medication or talk therapy to help you manage the depression, can help you get back to feeling like yourself again.

One study found that moms with postpartum depression are less likely to breastfeed their babies and are more likely to introduce cereal and other solid foods too early. These practices increase the risk of childhood obesity. However, if post-partum depression requires medication, it may be necessary to stop breastfeeding and switch to formula feeding, since some drugs migrate into breast milk. Do what's needed to help you feel better and bond better with your baby. Bonding with your baby is the most important consideration at this time.

To brighten your mental outlook and help you get back to your prepregnancy body weight, try to eat healthfully, exercise, and get plenty of fresh air and sunlight. Vitamin D is made in the skin by exposure to sunlight, and low levels of vitamin D have been linked to an increased risk of postpartum depression. For your mental health, try to go outside and get some sun. Exercising outdoors is especially helpful because it burns calories and tones muscles, and the sunlight helps your body make vitamin D.

To avoid sunburn, limit your exposure to about 20 minutes of sunlight a day, which is sufficient to boost vitamin D levels and improve mood. If you plan to stay outside for more than 20 minutes, be sure to apply sun protection lotion.

Effects of Stress and How to Cope

Too much stress, whether it's from worries about money, job, family or something else, is not good for you or your baby. In breastfeeding moms, stress interferes with milk production and milk let-down—the reflex that causes breast milk to be ejected into your baby's mouth when he sucks on the nipple.

For your baby, stress can disrupt brain development and cause behavioral problems. For you, stress is distracting and can prevent you from properly bonding with your baby. The effect on you can, in turn, trigger a stress response in your baby. The result is a vicious cycle that further undermines bonding between parent and child, which isn't good for your child's development and behavior.

Although some sources of stress may be out of your control, the way you cope with stress is within your control. Stress reduction techniques can help. For example, deep breathing, yoga or meditation can help you detach from your worries and focus on your baby. Religious or spiritual practices that calm or soothe you may be helpful. Breastfeeding and skin-to-skin contact can be soothing to you and your baby. Try to stay focused on your baby when you breastfeed, and enjoy the experience.

Daily physical activity such as brisk walking, or more strenuous exercise such as hiking or jogging, can reduce stress levels. The movement itself can reduce stress, but sometimes just being outside enjoying nature can allow you to view your worries from a fresh perspective.

If you sense that your stress level is becoming unmanageable, and you can't get the help you need from family or friends, be sure to seek professional help. Your baby needs your full attention at this critical period in his life.

Breastfeeding Moms Who Had Weight-Loss Surgery

Nearly 200,000 women in North America have weight-loss, or bariatric, surgery a year, and the number is increasing. This means that the number of babies born to women who had weight-loss surgery is also on the rise. Although data are scant, pregnancy often occurs during the first year after the surgery, when weight has not yet stabilized and the risk of nutritional deficiencies is greater.

Breastfeeding women who had weight-loss surgery often have a history of protein-calorie malnutrition or nutrient deficiencies in iron, calcium and many important vitamins including folic acid, vitamin D and vitamin K. Yet these are the building blocks for the tissues and organs of a baby and are also crucial for the development of the gut-brain partnership.

There's no doubt that taking prenatal vitamins during pregnancy is vitally important and may be advisable if you breastfeed your baby. Even more important is to eat a healthful variety of foods that provide proteins, healthy fats and carbohydrates, plus vitamins and minerals needed for your baby's developing brain.

If you had weight-loss surgery, the recommendations below will help ensure proper development of the baby's gut-brain partnership. See "The Gut-Brain Partnership: How It Affects Your Baby's Appetite and Weight" on page 20. This will guard against childhood obesity and help protect your own health:

- Breastfeeding is preferred. For additional support, contact a lactation consultant (visit *www.ilca.org*), or other qualified healthcare provider.

- Continue with your post-surgery visits to your doctor. Possible nutrient deficiencies should be carefully monitored and addressed as soon as possible.

- Visit a registered dietitian nutritionist to ensure your diet is varied and healthful and to obtain guidance on further weight loss, if needed.

- Discuss vitamin/mineral supplementation with your dietitian, doctor or qualified healthcare provider, including possible continued use of prenatal vitamins that include vitamin A as beta carotene, vitamin D, folic acid, vitamin B_{12}, iron, zinc, iodine and magnesium.

- Make sure your baby's pediatrician knows about your past surgery. Clinical evaluation and frequent monitoring of your baby's growth, by checking weight-for-length and head circumference, is especially important. Brain growth and development are rapidly occurring during infancy, and head circumference is a convenient way for the pediatrician to measure brain growth.

Breastfeeding Moms Who Are Vegans

If you're a vegan—a vegetarian who doesn't eat any animal foods—be sure to inform your baby's pediatrician, who can help make sure your breast milk contains the nutrients your baby needs. For example, a vegan diet lacks vitamin B_{12}, which can lead to anemia and abnormal brain and nerve development in your baby. A vegan mom must include a reliable source of vitamin B_{12} foods in her diet, such as fortified cereal and soymilk, and B_{12}-fortified nutritional yeast. If fortified foods are not eaten, a vitamin B_{12} supplement is recommended for mom.

It's very important that your baby's brain appetite centers grow properly, and your baby develops feeding behaviors that minimize the risk of childhood obesity. To help make this happen, it's essential that your baby gets sufficient amounts of the vitamins and minerals that play a crucial role in brain development, including folic acid, vitamin B_{12}, iron and zinc.

If you choose to eat vegan while breastfeeding, here are some key nutrients and foods to pay attention to.

Key Foods for Breastfeeding Vegans

Nutrient	Foods
Protein	Beans, chickpeas, edamame (green soybeans), nuts and nut butters, tofu and tempeh, seitan, quinoa, soymilk
Vitamin B_{12}	Fortified cereal, fortified soymilk, fortified nutritional yeast, vitamin B_{12} supplement
Vitamin D	Fortified soymilk and almond milk, fortified cereals, vitamin D supplement for breastfed infants (Note: Exposure of skin to sunlight makes vitamin D.)

Nutrient	Foods
Folic Acid (Folate)	Dark leafy green vegetables such as spinach, mustard greens, kale, collards Brussels sprouts, asparagus, broccoli, oranges, orange juice Beans and peas such as kidney beans, black-eyed peas, lentils Nuts, whole grains; grains with added folic acid, such as fortified cold cereals, enriched bread, pasta, rice
Iron	Beans and peas such as kidney beans, chickpeas, lentils Nuts and seeds such as almonds, cashews, pumpkin seeds, sunflower seeds Edamame, tofu, tempeh Whole grains, enriched grains Dark leafy green vegetables, dried fruits (Note: To increase iron absorption, eat foods containing iron along with foods rich in vitamin C such as berries, papaya, oranges, sweet peppers, broccoli and tomatoes.)
Zinc	Beans and peas such as navy beans, split peas, chickpeas, lentils Nuts and seeds such as almonds, cashews, walnuts, pumpkin seeds, sunflower seeds Tofu, tempeh Whole grains, wheat germ

Nutrient	Foods
Calcium	Tofu processed with calcium, fortified soymilk, soy yogurt Broccoli, kale, bok choy, collard greens, Chinese cabbage, okra Soybeans, almonds Calcium-fortified orange juice
Omega-3 Fatty Acid DHA	Foods fortified with DHA (from microalgae) such as DHA-fortified juice, soymilk, oils Vegan DHA supplement

Ask your baby's pediatrician if you should continue taking your prenatal supplement while breastfeeding. For additional dietary guidance, speak with a registered dietitian nutritionist.

Alcohol, Tobacco and Drugs

Drinking alcohol, smoking and taking street drugs are harmful to babies and may cause abnormal brain development. These toxins can also change the parents' behaviors and damage the interaction between parents and their baby.

For breastfeeding moms, alcohol, smoking and taking drugs can affect breast milk production and alter a baby's sleeping and eating behaviors. It's a myth that having a beer right before you breastfeed will increase your milk supply. Alcohol, as well as smoking, can actually reduce your milk supply since they lower the level of hormones that stimulate milk production and milk flow. Excessive drinking slows milk let-down, or the milk ejection reflex.

An occasional alcoholic drink may be OK, if the timing is right. Experts generally recommend that if a mom wants one alcoholic drink, she should wait about two to three hours to breastfeed after finishing her drink. This allows the alcohol levels in the breast milk to go down.

Alcohol and smoking can affect your baby's sleep. Research shows that in the 3.5 hours after breastfeeding, babies exposed to alcohol in breast milk spend less time sleeping and are less active when awake than babies not exposed to alcohol. Similarly, research on smoking has found that babies spend less time sleeping in the 3.5 hours after breastfeeding when their moms have recently smoked, and wake up from their naps sooner than babies of moms who don't smoke.

Smoking also causes nicotine to enter the breast milk. Secondhand smoke is not good for breastfed or formula-fed babies as it can lead to health problems such as asthma and bronchitis. Both smoking and secondhand smoke increase the risk of sudden infant death syndrome (SIDS). To help reduce the risks from smoke, make your home smoke free.

There's growing evidence that exposure to smoke from the mom or secondhand smoke from the dad may raise the risk of obesity in their children, particularly if smoking occurs during pregnancy. Although there's currently little research on the effect of parental smoking during infancy on childhood obesity, parents who smoke and would like to have more children should try to quit smoking before becoming pregnant again.

For your baby's health and future weight, live in a smoke-free home and avoid exposing your baby to secondhand smoke.

Most illegal and street drugs can enter the breast milk and reach the baby. These drugs can affect the baby's developing brain and nervous system and impair the parents' ability to take care of their baby. Moms who take illegal drugs should not breastfeed. If you take over-the-counter or prescription medications or herbal remedies, check with your doctor to make sure they're OK to take while breastfeeding.

Grandparents and Childhood Obesity

Grandparents are often a valuable source of support, as loving babysitters, substitute parents and concerned childcare advisors. Yet, grandparents, other relatives and friends are sometimes the source of outdated information on infant feeding and childrearing practices. Some well-meaning but mistaken advice may increase the chances of your child gaining excess weight. This includes introducing solid foods before your baby's 6 months old and adding infant cereal to a baby's bottle to help him sleep.

It's important that your child's doctor or healthcare provider monitors your child's weight-for-length and weight gain pattern and discusses family diet, activity and traditions that cover three generations of family. Taking steps to prevent childhood obesity now can help keep your child at a healthy weight as he gets older.

Keep in mind that research-based advice can change over time. Seek advice from qualified healthcare professionals who can assist you in keeping up with the latest research and practice. This will help you raise a healthy child in a way that works best for you and your family.

CHAPTER 10

In Summary

Much evidence suggests that the best time to prevent childhood obesity is during infancy and the first few years of life. This is when the brain is rapidly developing its appetite centers, and the communication between the gut and the brain—the gut-brain partnership—is also rapidly developing. It's possible to influence hunger and satiety, as well as taste preferences, during this period of your child's life.

Infancy is also a time when skin-to-skin contact can promote bonding with your baby, which reduces stress and fosters a sense of security and calm. Interacting with your young child and encouraging her to be physically active can guide her toward an active lifestyle. All of these factors can help your child stay at a healthy weight.

There's still much to learn about preventing obesity in children. Many factors raise the risk of obesity and some protect against it. Based on current science, a combination of the protective practices below will be most effective in keeping your baby at a healthy weight:

- Exclusively breastfeed your baby for at least the first six months of life.
- Introduce healthful solid foods after 6 months old.
- Pay attention to your baby's hunger and satiety cues to avoid overfeeding.

- Visit your baby's pediatrician, or a qualified healthcare provider, every two months to monitor your baby's rate of weight gain.

- Play (preferably outdoors) with your baby every day and encourage infant games.

- Skip the TV and screen time. Instead provide a safe space for your baby to explore and move around.

- Make sure your baby gets at least 12 hours of sleep each day.

- Avoid giving your baby sugary drinks and sweets.

One final thought: Prevention efforts during infancy can't guarantee your child will not grow up overweight or obese since the environment children live in encourages overeating, inactivity and not enough outdoor play. But parents can help their families beat these food and activity challenges. Building a strong foundation now is a solid investment in your baby's future health.

CHAPTER 11

Menu Plans (Introduction)

The Shape Up America!® dietitians and chef have created a weekly menu plan for breastfeeding and formula-feeding moms. Dads can use them too. These carefully-designed menus will help deliver the important nutrients that moms need to nourish themselves and their growing babies.

These menus meet the recommended servings from each food group for 2,300-calorie and 1,800-calorie meal plans. The menus focus on vegetables, fruits, whole grains, reduced-fat dairy and lean protein. They're also low in sugar.

Choosing the Right Calorie Levels

Moms who exclusively breastfeed will generally need a couple hundred calories more each day than moms who formula-feed or who breastfeed sometimes and also use formula.

Breastfeeding-only moms should aim for about 2,300 calories a day, using the menus found in Chapter 12 (page 113). Those looking to lose weight should keep to at least 1,800 calories a day for a healthy weight loss and to help ensure an adequate milk supply, using the menus found in Chapter 13 (page 121).

Formula-feeding moms or **breast-and-formula moms** can have about 1,800 calories a day, using the menus found in Chapter 13 (page 121); for weight loss, aim for about 1,400–1,600 calories a day.

Using the Menus

The menus include references to recipes, which we have collected in Chapter 14 (page 129). For nutrition facts, visit *www.shapeup.org* (enter the recipe name in the search box). For step-by-step directions with accompanying photographs, visit *www.shapeupfridge.com* (enter the recipe name in the search box).

Enjoy the menus as they are, or adapt them to fit your needs and food preferences. Visit *www.choosemyplate.gov/food-groups* for ideas on food swaps within each food group.

Remember, eating a variety of healthful foods is good for moms, dads and babies. Whether your baby's breastfed or formula fed, you're a role model for your family. Someday soon, when your baby reaches for the foods you're eating, make sure he chooses foods that are tasty and good for him.

Chapter 12

Menu Plans: 2,300 Calories

The menus in this chapter are appropriate for **breastfeeding-only moms who are not trying to lose weight**.

(If you are a breastfeeding-only mom looking to achieve healthy weight loss, or if you are not exclusively breastfeeding, consider the 1,800-calorie menus in Chapter 13, starting on page 121.)

For all menus, you should divide snacks throughout the day. You should also drink either water, an unsweetened flavored seltzer, or a no-calorie beverage throughout the day.

Day 1

Breakfast

- 1 cup toasted oats cereal sprinkled with 1 Tablespoon ground flaxseed
- 1 sliced banana
- 1 cup 1% milk (or unsweetened fortified soymilk)

Lunch

- **Veggie Tuna Salad** (page 134)
- 2 slices whole-wheat bread with 2 Tablespoons apple butter
- 2 small tangerines

Dinner

- 1 cantaloupe wedge
- 1 (4-ounce raw) skinless and boneless chicken breast, baked or grilled with 1 Tablespoon barbecue sauce
- 1 cup cooked broccoli florets with 1 teaspoon butter
- 1 baked sweet potato sprinkled with cinnamon
- 1 whole-wheat dinner roll
- 1 cup 1% milk (or unsweetened fortified soymilk)
- 1 fruit juice popsicle

Snacks

- ½ cup mixed dried fruit
- 3 cups air-popped popcorn with 1 teaspoon butter (or light microwave popcorn)
- 1 ounce nuts (about 10 walnut halves or 22 almonds or 35 shelled peanuts)
- Sugar-free hot cocoa prepared with 1 cup 1% milk (or unsweetened fortified soymilk)

Day 2

Breakfast

- **Strawberry Banana Smoothie** (page 140)
- 1 slice whole-wheat toast with 2 teaspoons natural peanut butter

Lunch

- **Chicken or Turkey Salad in Pita** (page 138)
- ½ avocado sprinkled with 1 teaspoon lemon juice
- 6 red and yellow bell pepper strips
- 1 medium pear

Dinner

- 1 serving **Tomato Peach Gazpacho** (page 140)
- 1 (4 ounces raw) flounder fillet cooked with 2 teaspoons olive oil, served with lemon wedge
- 1 cup cooked brown rice
- 1 cup cooked spinach sautéed with 2 chopped garlic cloves and 2 teaspoons olive oil
- 1 whole-wheat dinner roll
- ½ cup unsweetened applesauce sprinkled with cinnamon

Snacks

- 5 baby carrots with 1 Tablespoon light ranch salad dressing
- 2 rye crispbreads with 1 slice reduced-fat cheese
- 33 (1½ ounces) almonds
- 1 (6-ounce) container light yogurt, any flavor

Day 3

Breakfast

- 1 large cantaloupe wedge
- 2 slices whole-wheat toast with 1 Tablespoon natural peanut butter
- 1 cup 1% milk (or unsweetened fortified soymilk)

Lunch

- **Lean Roast Beef Sandwich** (page 138)
- 1 medium pear
- 2 Tablespoons unsalted roasted pumpkin seeds
- 1 cup 1% milk (or unsweetened fortified soymilk)

Dinner

- **Tossed Salad** (page 134)
- 1 serving **Grilled Shrimp and Pineapple with Citrus Glaze** (page 130)
- 1 cup cooked whole-wheat pasta with 1 teaspoon oil
- 1 fruit juice popsicle

Snacks

- 1 sliced banana mixed with 1 cup fat-free plain yogurt
- ¼ cup trail mix
- 8 unsalted three-ring pretzels

Day 4

Breakfast

- ½ cup calcium-fortified orange juice
- 1 cup cooked oatmeal with ½ cup blueberries
- 1 stick part-skim mozzarella string cheese
- 1 cup 1% milk (or unsweetened fortified soymilk)

Lunch

- 1 fast-food hamburger on bun
- 1 serving side salad with 1 Tablespoon regular salad dressing
- 1 serving fast-food apple slices
- 1 serving fruit and low-fat yogurt parfait

Dinner

- ½ cup low-sodium tomato or vegetable juice
- 1 serving **Stuffed Eggplant Spears** (page 131)
- 1 serving **Tabuli** (page 136)
- 1 whole-wheat dinner roll
- ¼ cup dried fruit and nut mix

Snacks

- 6 baby carrots
- ½ cup low-fat cottage cheese mixed with ½ cup canned pineapple packed in its own juice
- 1 sandwich made with 2 slices whole-wheat bread, 1½ Tablespoons natural peanut butter and 1 Tablespoon spreadable fruit
- 1 cup 1% milk (or unsweetened fortified soymilk)

Day 5

Breakfast

- ½ grapefruit
- 2 eggs cooked with nonstick cooking spray
- 2 slices whole-wheat toast with 1 Tablespoon apple butter
- 1 cup 1% milk (or unsweetened fortified soymilk)

Lunch

- **Chicken Sandwich** (page 139)
- 6 baby carrots
- 1 large banana
- 1 cup 1% milk (or unsweetened fortified soymilk)

Dinner

- **Spinach Salad** (page 135)
- 1 serving **Grilled Salmon** (page 132)
- 1 serving **Farro Spring Salad** (page 137)
- 1 whole-wheat dinner roll
- 1 cup cantaloupe chunks
- 1 cup 1% milk (or unsweetened fortified soymilk)

Snacks

- 1 cup plain nonfat yogurt mixed with 1 miniature box raisins and 6 walnut halves
- 3 cups air-popped popcorn with 1 teaspoon melted butter and sprinkled with seasoning (cinammon, garlic powder, chili powder, or a no-salt seasoning blend); or use light microwave popcorn
- 2 large graham crackers (4 squares)

Day 6

Breakfast

- ½ cup calcium-fortified orange juice
- 1 cup bran flakes
- 1 sliced banana
- 1 cup 1% milk (or unsweetened fortified soymilk)

Lunch

- **Cheese Sandwich** (page 139)
- 6 red and yellow bell pepper strips
- 1 medium apple
- 1 cup 1% milk (or unsweetened fortified soymilk)

Dinner

- **Tossed Salad** (page 134)
- 1 broiled pork chop (5 ounces raw with bone)
- ¾ cup cooked couscous (¼ cup dry)
- ½ cup canned no-salt-added stewed tomatoes
- 1 whole-wheat dinner roll
- 1 serving **Flat Peach Pie** (page 141)

Snacks

- ½ cup grapes (or freeze the grapes)
- 1 ounce nuts (about 10 walnut halves or 22 almonds or 35 shelled peanuts)
- 1 (6-ounce) container fat-free plain or light yogurt

Day 7

Breakfast

- ½ cup calcium-fortified orange juice
- 2 scrambled eggs cooked with 1 teaspoon vegetable oil
- 2 slices toasted whole-wheat bread with 1 Tablespoon natural peanut butter
- 1 cup 1% milk (or unsweetened fortified soymilk)

Lunch

- **Pita Melt** (page 139)
- 1 ounce (about 16) baked tortilla chips with 2 Tablespoons guacamole
- 1 medium peach
- 1 cup 1% milk (or unsweetened fortified soymilk)

Dinner

- 1 cup low sodium tomato or vegetable juice
- 1 serving **Light Chili** (page 133)
- **Mixed Green Salad** (page 135)
- 1 cup cooked brown rice
- 1 medium wedge (or 2 cups cubed) watermelon

Snacks

- 1 orange
- 1 cup fat-free plain yogurt mixed with 1 miniature box raisins
- 3 cups air-popped popcorn or one 100-calorie microwave popcorn bag

Chapter 13

Menu Plans: 1,800 Calories

The menu plans in this chapter are appropriate for **two groups:** breastfeeding-only moms who are trying to achieve healthy weight loss, and moms who are not exclusively breastfeeding.

(If you are a breastfeeding-only mom who is not attempting to lose weight, use the 2,300-calorie menus in Chapter 12, starting on page 113.)

For all menus, you should divide snacks throughout the day. You should also drink either water, an unsweetened flavored seltzer, or a no-calorie beverage throughout the day.

Day 1

Breakfast

- 1 cup toasted oats cereal sprinkled with 1 Tablespoon ground flaxseed
- 1 sliced banana
- 1 cup 1% milk (or unsweetened fortified soymilk)

Lunch

- **Veggie Tuna Salad** (page 134)
- 1 slice whole-wheat bread with 2 teaspoons apple butter
- 2 small tangerines

Dinner

- 1 cantaloupe wedge
- 1 (4-ounce raw) skinless and boneless chicken breast, baked or grilled with 1 Tablespoon barbecue sauce
- 1 cup cooked broccoli florets
- 1 baked sweet potato sprinkled with cinnamon
- 1 whole-wheat dinner roll
- 1 cup 1% milk (or unsweetened fortified soymilk)

Snacks

- 3 cups air-popped popcorn or light microwave popcorn
- 1 ounce nuts (about 10 walnut halves or 22 almonds or 35 shelled peanuts)
- Sugar-free hot cocoa prepared with 1 cup 1% milk (or unsweetened fortified soymilk)

Day 2

Breakfast

- **Strawberry Banana Smoothie** (page 140)

Lunch

- **Chicken or Turkey Salad in Pita** (page 138)
- 6 red and yellow bell pepper strips
- 1 medium pear

Dinner

- 1 serving **Tomato Peach Gazpacho** (page 140)
- 1 (4-ounce raw) flounder fillet cooked with 2 teaspoons olive oil, served with lemon wedge
- 1 cup cooked brown rice
- 1 cup cooked spinach sautéed with 2 chopped garlic cloves and ½ Tablespoon olive oil
- 1 whole-wheat dinner roll
- ½ cup unsweetened applesauce sprinkled with cinnamon

Snacks

- 5 baby carrots with 1 Tablespoon light ranch salad dressing
- 1 rye crispbread with 1 slice (1 ounce) reduced-fat cheese
- 22 (1 ounce) almonds
- 1 (6-ounce) container light yogurt, any flavor

Day 3

Breakfast

- 1 cantaloupe wedge
- 2 slices whole-wheat toast with 1 Tablespoon natural peanut butter
- 1 cup 1% milk (or unsweetened fortified soymilk)

Lunch

- **Lean Roast Beef Sandwich** (page 138)
- 1 medium pear
- 1 cup 1% milk (or unsweetened fortified soymilk)

Dinner

- **Tossed Salad** (page 134)
- 1 serving **Grilled Shrimp and Pineapple with Citrus Glaze** (page 130)
- 1 cup cooked whole-wheat pasta with 1 teaspoon oil
- 1 fruit juice popsicle

Snacks

- 1 sliced banana mixed with 1 cup fat-free plain yogurt
- 5 unsalted three-ring pretzels

Day 4

Breakfast

- ½ cup calcium-fortified orange juice
- 1 cup cooked oatmeal with ½ cup blueberries
- 1 stick part-skim mozzarella string cheese
- 1 cup 1% milk (or unsweetened fortified soymilk)

Lunch

- 1 fast-food hamburger on bun
- 1 serving side salad with 1 Tablespoon regular salad dressing
- 1 serving fast-food apple slices
- 1 serving fruit and low-fat yogurt parfait

Dinner

- 1 cup low-sodium tomato or vegetable juice
- 1 serving **Stuffed Eggplant Spears** (page 131)
- 1 serving **Tabuli** (page 136)
- 1 whole-wheat dinner roll
- ¼ cup dried fruit and nut mix

Snacks

- 6 baby carrots with 1 Tablespoon hummus
- ½ cup low-fat cottage cheese mixed with ½ cup canned pineapple packed in its own juice
- ½ sandwich made with 1 slice whole-wheat bread, ½ Tablespoon natural peanut butter and 1 Tablespoon spreadable fruit
- 1 cup 1% milk (or unsweetened fortified soymilk)

Day 5

Breakfast

- ½ grapefruit
- 1 egg cooked with nonstick cooking spray
- 1 slice whole-wheat toast with 2 teaspoons apple butter
- 1 cup 1% milk (or unsweetened fortified soymilk)

Lunch

- **Chicken Sandwich** (page 139)
- 6 baby carrots
- 1 medium banana
- 1 cup 1% milk (or unsweetened fortified soymilk)

Dinner

- **Spinach Salad** (page 135)
- 1 serving **Grilled Salmon** (page 132)
- 1 serving **Farro Spring Salad** (page 137)
- 1 cup cantaloupe chunks

Snacks

- 1 cup plain nonfat yogurt mixed with 1 miniature box raisins
- 3 cups air-popped popcorn with 1 teaspoon melted butter and sprinkled with seasoning (cinammon, garlic powder, chili powder, or a no-salt seasoning blend); or use light microwave popcorn
- 1 large graham cracker (2 squares)

Day 6

Breakfast

- 1 cup bran flakes
- 1 sliced banana
- 1 cup 1% milk (or unsweetened fortified soymilk)

Lunch

- **Cheese Sandwich** (page 139)
- 6 red and yellow bell pepper strips
- 1 medium apple

Dinner

- **Tossed Salad** (page 134)
- 1 broiled pork chop (5 ounces raw with bone)
- 1 cup cooked couscous (⅓ cup dry)
- ½ cup canned no-salt-added stewed tomatoes
- 1 serving **Flat Peach Pie** (page 141)

Snacks

- ½ cup grapes (or freeze the grapes)
- 5 whole-wheat crackers
- 1 ounce nuts (about 10 walnut halves or 22 almonds or 35 shelled peanuts)
- 1 (6-ounce) container fat-free plain or light yogurt

Day 7

Breakfast

- 1 scrambled egg cooked with 1 teaspoon vegetable oil
- 2 slices toasted whole-wheat bread with 1 Tablespoon natural peanut butter
- 1 cup 1% milk (or unsweetened fortified soymilk)

Lunch

- **Pita Melt** (page 139)
- 1 ounce (about 16) baked tortilla chips with 2 Tablespoons guacamole
- 1 medium peach
- 1 cup 1% milk (or unsweetened fortified soymilk)

Dinner

- 1 cup low sodium tomato or vegetable juice
- 1 serving **Light Chili** (page 133)
- **Mixed Green Salad** (page 135)
- ½ cup cooked brown rice
- 1 cup cubed watermelon

Snacks

- 1 orange
- 3 cups air-popped popcorn or one 100-calorie microwave popcorn bag

CHAPTER 14

Recipes

This chapter contains the basic directions for the recipes used in the menu plans of Chapter 12 (page 113) and Chapter 13 (page 121).

Nutrition facts can be found at *www.shapeup.org* (enter the recipe name in the search box).

For step-by-step recipe directions with accompanying photographs, visit *www.shapeupfridge.com* (enter the recipe name in the search box).

Grilled Shrimp and Pineapple with Citrus Glaze

Serves 4

Ingredients

    1 pound large shrimp, peeled and deveined, fresh or frozen

    ½ fresh pineapple

    ½ cup mushrooms, halved

    ½ cup water

    6 Tablespoons orange marmalade

    1 Tablespoon reduced sodium soy sauce

    ½ jalapeno (optional)

Directions

1. Defrost shrimp in cold water if needed, drain and pat dry, or rinse and pat dry fresh shrimp.

2. Core and slice the pineapple into 16 chunks, or similar size to the shrimp.

3. Cut the mushrooms in half.

4. If using wooden skewers, soak in water for about 5 minutes. Then skewer the shrimp, pineapple, and mushrooms, using about 4 shrimp per skewer.

5. Make the citrus glaze by combining the water, orange marmalade, soy sauce, and jalapeno (optional) in a small pot. Warm briefly and whisk just to dissolve marmalade.

6. Before grilling, brush the skewers with the citrus glaze. Grill the shrimp for 3–5 minutes on the grill, or until the shrimp just turns pink.

7. When the skewers are done, heat the citrus glaze and bring to a boil. Serve the skewers with a side of the citrus glaze.

Stuffed Eggplant Spears

Serves 6 (2 spears each)

Ingredients

2 large eggplants

¼ cup olive oil, divided in half

3 cloves garlic, minced

½ onion, sliced

1 red or green bell pepper, or combination of both, cut in 1-inch strips

2 tomatoes, chopped

1 can (8 ounces) no salt added tomato sauce, divided in half

⅛ teaspoon salt and pepper

parsley (for garnish)

Directions

1. Preheat the oven to 450°F. Wash and cut the eggplants in half, then each half in thirds. You should end with 12 eggplant spears in total. Place the eggplant spears on a baking tray and brush with 2 Tablespoons olive oil. Place in the oven for 15–20 minutes, or until fork tender.

2. While eggplants are baking, prepare the filling. Chop the garlic, onions, bell pepper, and tomatoes. In a medium to large sauté pan, heat 2 Tablespoons olive oil and place all garlic, onions, and peppers on medium heat for 5–7 minutes, or until onions become tender. Then add tomatoes and cook another 2–3 minutes or until most liquid has evaporated. Set aside to cool.

3. When the eggplants are done, place them in a 13" x 9" baking dish. Slice each eggplant spear vertically with a fork and knife, being careful not to cut through the skin. Pry open and fill with 2–3 Tablespoons filling.

4. Cover stuffed eggplant with half of the tomato sauce. Either cover with plastic wrap and place in the refrigerator overnight, or set oven to 350°F to bake. Before serving, uncover plastic wrap, place the remaining tomato sauce on eggplant and bake at 350°F for 30 minutes. Garnish with snipped parsley.

Grilled Salmon

Serves 6

Ingredients

1–1½ pounds salmon fillet

⅛ teaspoon salt

⅛ teaspoon freshly cracked pepper

cooking spray

Directions

1. With a very sharp knife, portion the salmon fillet into 6 equal pieces, or ask your fishmonger to do this for you. Leave the skin on to keep its shape.

2. Sprinkle the salmon fillets with salt and pepper.

3. Spray a heated grill. When the grill is almost smoking, place fillets on grill. Cook 3–4 minutes per side, depending on your preferred degree of doneness. Turn the salmon on its side to grill for a brief 1–2 minutes if the temperature is very high, to make sure the salmon gets cooked throughout. Cooking time may vary depending on the temperature of your grill and thickness of the fillets. Pinch salmon; a firm pinch in the middle of the fillet will mean it's medium-well done. It will continue to cook after it's removed from the grill.

Light Chili

Serves 7

Ingredients

1 teaspoon vegetable oil

2 ounces Canadian bacon, diced small

1 large onion, finely chopped

2 large garlic cloves, peeled and minced

1 pound lean ground beef (96% lean) or lean ground turkey

1 Tablespoon plus 1½ teaspoons chili powder

1½ teaspoon ground cumin

1½ teaspoon paprika

½–1½ teaspoons cayenne pepper

1 can (14.5 ounces) crushed tomatoes (fire-roasted or regular)

1 can (8 ounces) tomato sauce

1½ cups low-sodium beef stock

1 teaspoon Worcestershire sauce

2 cans (14.5 ounces each) low-sodium black beans, drained

low-fat sour cream, sliced scallions, and/or grated low-sodium cheddar cheese for topping

Directions

1. In a large pot over medium heat, add the oil. Once hot, add the Canadian bacon and onions and cook just until onions and bacon begin to brown, about 4 minutes. Stir while cooking. Then lower heat, stir in the garlic and cook 1 minute.

2. Increase the heat to medium-high and add ground beef or turkey. Break up the meat with a spoon and stir gently until it loses its pink color, 6–8 minutes. Stir in the spices, tomatoes, tomato sauce, beef stock, and Worcestershire sauce. Bring mixture to a boil. Reduce heat to medium-low, cover partially and cook 30 minutes.

3. Add drained beans and cook 10 minutes, uncovered. Serve warm, with toppings (sour cream, scallions, and/or grated cheese) on the side.

Veggie Tuna Salad

Ingredients

>   2 cups leafy greens (romaine, red or green leaf lettuce)
>   chopped red bell pepper
>   sliced cucumber
>   cherry tomatoes
>   1 Tablespoon olive oil
>   1 teaspoon vinegar
>   1 small (3-ounce) can water-packed light tuna
>   1 Tablespoon light mayonnaise

Directions

1. Toss greens, red pepper, cucumber and tomatoes all together with oil and vinegar.

2. Mix tuna with light mayonnaise; spoon on top of tossed veggies.

Tossed Salad

Ingredients

>   2 cups romaine lettuce
>   sliced red bell pepper
>   sliced cucumber
>   cherry tomatoes
>   1 Tablespoon olive oil
>   1 teaspoon vinegar

Directions

1. Toss all ingredients together and serve.

Spinach Salad

Ingredients

> 2 cups spinach
> sliced mushrooms
> sliced red onion
> 1 Tablespoon olive oil
> 1 teaspoon vinegar

Directions

1. Toss all ingredients together and serve.

Mixed Green Salad

Ingredients

> 2 cups mixed greens
> 2 Tablespoons (½-ounce) slivered almonds
> 1 Tablespoon olive oil
> 1 teaspoon vinegar

Directions

1. Toss all ingredients together and serve.

Tabuli

Serves 6 (¾ cup each)

Ingredients

    1 cup fine or small bulgur wheat

2–3 cups water

    1 cup finely chopped green onions (scallions)

    1 cup finely chopped mint

    1 cup finely chopped parsley

    ⅓ cup extra virgin olive oil

    1 lemon (approx.) to yield ¼ cup juice

2–3 tomatoes, finely diced (optional)

½–1 cucumber finely diced (optional)

½–1 teaspoon salt

    freshly cracked pepper

Directions

1. Add 1 cup fine bulgur into a large serving bowl. Add water until bulgur is just covered. Let sit for 30 minutes until almost all water is absorbed. If water is not all absorbed after 30 minutes, hold a paper towel over bowl tightly and drain. If all water is absorbed before 30 minutes, add more water to keep bulgur moist.

2. While bulgur is soaking, chop all herbs and vegetables. Mix the olive oil and lemon juice.

3. When bulgur is ready, add herbs, vegetables, and dressing, and salt and pepper to taste. Top with halved cherry tomatoes if desired.

Farro Spring Salad

Serves 7

Ingredients

5 cups water

1 cup raw farro

¼ teaspoon salt

1 small bunch asparagus, or 8 large asparagus spears

2 carrots

¼ onion

4 Tablespoons extra virgin olive oil

4 Tablespoons lemon juice + zest of 1 lemon

4 Tablespoons mint, chopped

4 Tablespoons parsley, chopped

¼ cup halved cherry tomatoes

⅛ teaspoon freshly cracked pepper

3 Tablespoons feta crumbles (optional)

Directions

1. Bring 5 cups water to a boil in a medium saucepan, then add farro and salt. Bring back to a boil then simmer 30 minutes. Let the farro sit for 5 minutes or until tender. Drain in a colander. Then, place farro in a salad bowl serving dish.

2. Peel the tough ends of the asparagus and trim the stems. Using a mandolin or vegetable peel, peel ribbons and set aside. Do the same for the carrots. Slice onion thinly and place in cold water (to tone down flavor).

3. In the same pot you used to cook farro, fill with water and bring to a boil. Have an ice bath or cold water bath on standby. Blanch, or dunk asparagus in boiling water for 10–30 seconds, then place in ice bath. Repeat with carrots. Drain, then add to farro in serving dish.

4. To make the dressing, add the olive oil, lemon juice and zest, and stir well. Pour dressing over the salad. Add chopped mint, parsley, onions, tomatoes, pepper, and feta. Mix well. Serve at room temperature or as a cold salad.

Chicken or Turkey Salad in Pita

Ingredients

    ½ cup chicken or turkey salad

    1 Tablespoon light mayonnaise

      lettuce

      sliced tomato

    1 large whole-wheat pita

Directions

1. Mix chicken or turkey salad with mayonnaise, lettuce and tomato.

2. Fill pita and serve.

Lean Roast Beef Sandwich

Ingredients

    2 slices rye bread

    2 teaspoons spicy mustard

    3 (1 ounce each) slices lean deli roast beef

    1 romaine lettuce leaf

      sliced onion

      sliced tomato

Directions

1. Spread mustard on rye bread; top with beef, lettuce, onion and tomato; serve.

Chicken Sandwich

Ingredients

> 1 whole-wheat bun
> 1 Tablespoon light mayonnaise
> 3 ounces baked or grilled skinless chicken breast
>   sliced tomato

Directions

> **1.** Spread bun with mayonnaise; top with chicken and tomato; serve.

Cheese Sandwich

Ingredients

> 2 slices whole-wheat bread
> 1 teaspoon mustard
> 2 (1 ounce each) slices reduced-fat cheese
>   sliced tomato
>   oregano or basil (optional, for seasoning)

Directions

> **1.** Spread mustard on bread; top with cheese, tomato and seasoning; serve.

Pita Melt

Ingredients

> 1 cup sliced raw vegetables (e.g., zucchini, broccoli, mushrooms, bell peppers)
> 1 medium whole wheat pita
> ½ cup shredded reduced-fat cheese

Directions

> **1.** Microwave vegetables 1–2 minutes, or until tender.
> **2.** Put vegetables in pita and top with cheese.
> **3.** Place pita in microwave for 1-2 minutes, or until cheese melts; serve.

Tomato Peach Gazpacho

Serves 4

Ingredients

>   1 heirloom tomato
>   1 flat peach
>   1 sliver of yellow chile pepper (optional)
>   ¼ teaspoon salt
>   2 teaspoons extra virgin olive oil
>   1–2 Tablespoons chopped chives or scallions

Directions

1. Blend all ingredients except chives or scallions in a food processor, immersion blender, or stand blender until liquid. Store in the refrigerator for at least 2 hours before serving (or chill tomato and peach in refrigerator before blending for immediate service). Garnish with chopped chives or scallions before serving.

Strawberry Banana Smoothie

Ingredients

>   ½ cup (about 6) frozen unsweetened strawberries*
>   1 medium banana
>   1 cup 1% milk (or unsweetened fortified soymilk)
>   ½ cup plain fat-free Greek yogurt
>   1 teaspoon sugar or no-calorie sweetener (to taste)

* Optionally, substitute fresh strawberries plus 4–5 ice cubes

Directions

1. Combine and blend all ingredients in blender; serve.

Flat Peach Pie

Serves 1

Ingredients

    1 flat peach

    2 Tablespoons fat-free vanilla Greek frozen yogurt

    2 raspberries for garnish

    5 almonds for garnish

    ½ teaspoon ground cinnamon

Directions

1. Set the oven to 400°F.

2. Place the peach on a small non-stick pan and put in the oven for 15 minutes or until the peach is slightly soft.

3. Serve hot topped with the frozen yogurt. Use raspberries and almonds as the garnish, with a sprinkle of cinnamon.

Appendix A

Glossary

AAP (American Academy of Pediatrics)
A professional organization of 60,000 pediatricians dedicated to the health, safety, and well-being of infants, children, adolescents and young adults. The FAAP designation after a pediatrician's name stands for Fellow of the American Academy of Pediatrics. Pediatricians who use FAAP have obtained initial board certification in pediatrics.

Agility
The ability to change the body's position or direction quickly and easily.

Amniotic fluid
The fluid that completely surrounds the developing fetus in a mother's womb.

Antibiotics
Compounds that are capable of killing bacteria. Although antibiotics are usually targeted to kill harmful bacteria, they can also kill beneficial bacteria, possibly upsetting the balance between beneficial bacteria and harmful bacteria that live in the intestines of mammals, including humans.

Appetite centers
Specific regions of the brain that are known to influence appetite. There are appetite centers in the hypothalamus and brainstem. The appetite centers are turned on or off by nutrient, hormonal and nerve signals coming from the gut. The appetite centers affect the amount of food eaten by influencing when a meal starts, how long it lasts and when it ends. The appetite centers consist of hunger and satiety centers.

The hunger center is the region of the brain that senses the hormonal and nerve signals that hunger is developing. When the hunger signals become strong enough, the brain directs changes in feeding behavior. In an infant, behavioral signals such as rooting for the nipple, sucking, being fussy or crying will signal hunger.

The satiety center is the region of the brain that senses the nutrient, hormonal and nerve signals that satiety, or fullness, is developing. When the satiety signals become strong enough, the brain directs changes in feeding behavior. Infants may suck less vigorously, turn their head away, or become annoyed or drowsy, which signals that the meal is over.

Baby-friendly hospital

A designation set by WHO for hospitals that meet all 10 criteria for promoting breastfeeding. The Baby-friendly Hospital Initiative (BFHI) was launched by WHO and UNICEF (United Nations Children's Fund). It is a global effort to implement practices that protect, promote and support breastfeeding, with 152 countries, including the U.S., participating.

BMI (body mass index)

A ratio of a person's weight to height; determined by dividing weight (in kilograms) by the square of height (in meters), or kg/m^2. There are no BMI standards in younger children, so BMI isn't used until age 2. In infants, weight and recumbent length, which is the length of the baby lying down and facing up, are measured to track growth. The relationship of weight to length is compared to a reference standard based on the growth of a very large number of healthy babies from diverse racial and ethnic backgrounds. There are separate standards for boys and girls since their growth patterns differ.

CDC (Centers for Disease Control and Prevention)

A government agency that is part of the Department of Health and Human Services. It protects Americans from health, safety and security threats that originate abroad and in the U.S. Within the CDC, the Division of Nutrition, Physical Activity and Obesity leads public health efforts to prevent and control obesity, chronic disease and other health conditions through regular physical activity and good nutrition.

Clostridium botulinum

Dangerous bacteria that can cause a serious, sometimes fatal, illness called botulism. They are sometimes present as spores in honey and can multiply in the gastrointestinal tract of an infant and potentially cause life-threatening botulism. For this reason, honey should not be fed to infants. Although a baby's intestinal tract is unable to destroy these harmful bacteria, an older child's intestinal tract is able to prevent the growth of these spores and their toxin.

Colostrum

The fluid secreted by the mother's breasts during the first week of the baby's life, before her regular milk comes in. Colostrum is rich in antibodies, nutrients, and growth factors and contains hormones such as leptin and ghrelin, which are involved in feeding behavior.

Demand feeding

Also called responsive feeding, in which the baby is fed when he starts signaling that he is hungry. *See also: scheduled feeding.*

Exclusive breastfeeding

A practice of feeding only breast milk, which is recommended by the AAP for the first six months of life. It means no formula, water, juice, soda or pop, sugar water, honey, fruit drinks or infant cereal in a bowl or added to the bottle.

Expressed breast milk

Milk that is taken from the breast either manually or with a breast pump.

Foremilk

The first milk produced by the breast when a baby starts feeding. It's different in composition and taste from the hindmilk produced by the breast at the end of the meal. *See also: hindmilk.*

Genes

The basic unit of heredity. Every cell contains a set of genes, made up of DNA, which determines the development and characteristics of the body. For example, your genes will dictate the color of your eyes.

Genetic expression

A process that uses information in your genes, which is stored in a molecule called DNA, to make the gene product RNA. The RNA serves as a blueprint for manufacturing proteins produced by the cell. Many factors affect the expression of the DNA that makes up the genes. This includes diet, stress and environmental chemicals. These factors determine whether a person's genes are turned on or off, and if they are turned on, the degree to which they function. For example, diet influences the genetic expression of height. Genes will dictate how tall a person can become, but if the diet is poor when a child is growing, the child will not reach his full height.

Genetics

The branch of biology that focuses on the study of genes and heredity. It explains how traits are inherited during conception and expressed during development.

Ghrelin

A gut hormone that signals hunger to the brain. It's also found in human breast milk. Ghrelin is often called the hunger hormone.

Gastrointestinal tract

The digestive tract, also called the GI tract, which includes the stomach, small intestine and large intestine. *See also: gut.*

Gross motor skills

Skills that use large muscle groups, such as the arms and legs, to enable the body to move. Gross motor skills that babies develop include rolling over, sitting up, crawling and walking.

Gut

Part of the body that consists of the gastrointestinal tract, pancreas, liver and associated fat (adipose) tissue. Nutrient, hormonal and nerve signals go from the gut to the brain to signal the development of hunger or satiety. *See also: gastrointestinal tract.*

Gut-brain partnership

The system in which the gut and brain communicate with each other to signal either hunger or satiety. This communication determines eating behavior, including the start and end of a meal, how long the meal lasts, and how many meals are eaten, which all affect how much food is eaten.

Hindmilk

The milk produced by the mother's breast toward the end of the meal when a baby is feeding. It's different in composition and taste from the foremilk produced by the breast at the start of the meal. Some of the changes in the composition of hindmilk promote satiety in the infant. *See also: foremilk.*

Hunger

An unpleasant sensation from a lack of food that leads to a desire to eat. It's a component of appetite that's the opposite of satiety. A sensation of hunger develops within hours after eating a meal and strengthens as hormonal and nerve signals monitor a decrease in energy stores or nutrients. *See also: satiety and appetite centers.*

IOM (Institute of Medicine)

An independent, nonprofit organization that works outside of the U.S. government to provide unbiased and authoritative advice to decision makers and the public. It's the health arm of the National Academy of Sciences and addresses questions about the nation's health and healthcare.

Leptin

A gut hormone that signals satiety to the brain. It's also found in human breast milk and colostrum. Leptin is often called the satiety hormone.

Milk let-down

A reflex that releases milk stored in the breast and ejects it into the milk ducts so it flows into the baby's mouth. The baby's sucking on the nipple stimulates milk let-down. Factors that may interfere with let-down include fatigue, stress and pain.

NCHS (National Center for Health Statistics)

A division of the CDC that collects data on vital health statistics of Americans. The statistical information is used to identify and address health issues and help guide public health and health policy decisions.

Neophobia

"Neo" means new and "phobia" means fear. Food neophobia is a reluctance or unwillingness of children, including infants, to try new foods.

Normal

A term used in statistics to describe the distribution of measurements of a population. For example, measured height and weight are used to create tables and growth curves that describe normal growth of infants and children. This allows the growth pattern of a baby to be compared to many thousands of healthy babies of the same age and sex.

Obesity

An excessive amount of weight in the form of fat that raises the risk of diseases such as diabetes, heart disease, sleep apnea and certain cancers. In adults, obesity is defined as a body mass index (BMI) of 30.0 or higher. In children, obesity is defined as a weight-for-length at the 95th percentile or higher. However, this definition may not detect obesity developing in children of normal weight who are gaining weight rapidly but whose weight-for-length still falls within the normal range. For this reason, frequent monitoring by a pediatric healthcare professional and keeping an accurate and complete history of weight-for-length records on each child are important to prevent childhood obesity. *See also: overweight.*

Overweight

The accumulation of excess weight in the form of fat that may signal the developing possibility of obesity. In adults, overweight is defined as a body mass index (BMI) of 25.0 to 29.9. In children, overweight is defined as a weight-for-length at the 85th percentile to less than the 95th percentile. However, this definition of overweight may not detect the accumulation of excess fat in children who are gaining weight rapidly but whose weight-for-length still falls within the normal range. For this reason, frequent monitoring by a pediatric healthcare professional and keeping an accurate and complete history of weight-for-length records on each child are important to prevent childhood obesity. *See also: obesity.*

Percentile

A statistical term that can be applied to height, weight, head circumference or any other measurement related to a child's growth. The percentiles in growth charts are based on a large reference population of healthy children. They allow pediatricians to track and compare the growth of a single child to that of other children of the same age and sex. For example, if a child's height is at the 30th percentile, it means that 30 percent of children his age and sex are shorter and 70 percent are taller. If a child's weight is at the 95th percentile, it means that 95 percent of children his age and sex weigh less and 5 percent weigh more than this child.

Recumbent length

A measure taken of a baby's length while lying down and facing up. Since babies cannot stand, recumbent length is used instead of height to track their growth.

Rooming-in

A hospital policy that allows a newborn baby to stay with the mother 24 hours a day, from the moment of birth to the time they leave the hospital.

Rooting reflex

An instinctual movement in which a baby will turn his head from side to side looking for the nipple. When a hungry baby's cheek or lips are touched, the baby will make sucking, or rooting motions with his mouth.

Satiety

A feeling of fullness; the opposite of hunger. It's the result of nutrient, hormonal and nerve signals that develop and strengthen during a meal. Once a meal ends, satiety prevents further eating until hunger returns. *See also: hunger and appetite centers.*

Scheduled feeding

The practice of feeding a baby on a schedule set by someone other than the baby. In a hospital, the nursing staff may set the schedule. A working mother may find it more practical to have the baby adapt to a feeding schedule that she or a caregiver sets. *See also: demand feeding.*

Shaken baby syndrome

A type of inflicted brain injury that happens when a baby is violently shaken. It's a severe and preventable form of child abuse that can cause blindness, seizures, brain damage or death.

SIDS (sudden infant death syndrome)

The sudden death of an infant under one year of age, which cannot be explained after a thorough investigation is conducted.

Weaning

The gradual process of introducing solid foods, usually one at a time with several days to one week between each new food. The AAP recommends delaying weaning until the baby is 6 months old and developmentally ready for solid foods. This can help prevent childhood obesity. Discuss with your baby's pediatrician when it's best to start weaning.

WHO (World Health Organization)

The authority for health within the United Nations system. Based in Geneva, Switzerland, its responsibilities include providing leadership on global health matters, health research and evidence-based policy, and monitoring and assessing health trends.

Appendix B

Resources

Breastfeeding Videos, Resources and Helpline

womenshealth.gov

Website by the Office on Women's Health (OWH) of the U.S. Department of Health and Human Services that provides accurate information on the health of women. The website includes comprehensive information on breastfeeding.

Breastfeeding advice, videos and information are available at:

www.womenshealth.gov/breastfeeding/
finding-support-and-information/videos.html

Help with learning how to breastfeed can be found at:

www.womenshealth.gov/breastfeeding/learning-to-breastfeed/#d

Advice for pumping and milk storage can be found at:

www.womenshealth.gov/breastfeeding/pumping-and-milk-storage

The number for the National Breastfeeding Helpline is 1-800-994-9662.

International Lactation Consultant Association (ILCA)

Find a certified lactation consultant near you by visiting *www.ilca.org*.

La Leche League International

Visit *www.llli.org* for information and support for breastfeeding moms, including answers to breastfeeding questions such as nursing multiples; mother-to-mother forums; breastfeeding and the law; and an online magazine *Breastfeeding Today*.

North Carolina Breastfeeding Coalition

Visit *www.ncbfc.org* for information for parents on breastfeeding in public and the workplace, as well as on storing and expressing human milk.

Books

American Academy of Pediatrics New Mother's Guide to Breastfeeding. Joan Younger Meek, editor in chief. New York: Bantam Books; 2011.

A Parent's Guide to Childhood Obesity: A Road Map to Health. Sandra G. Hassink, editor in chief. Elk Grove Village, IL: American Academy of Pediatrics; 2006.

Baby Builders: An Exercise Program for Stronger Healthier Babies. Jenna Zervas. Branson, MO: Developing By Design; 2006.

Eating Expectantly: Practical Advice for Healthy Eating Before, During and After Pregnancy. 4th ed. Bridget Swinney. El Paso, TX: Healthy Food Zone Media; 2013.

Fearless Feeding: How to Raise Healthy Eaters from High Chair to High School. Jill Castle and Maryann Jacobsen. San Francisco, CA: Jossey-Bass; 2013.

Nutrition: What Every Parent Needs to Know. 2nd ed. William H. Dietz and Loraine Stern, eds. Elk Grove Village, IL: American Academy of Pediatrics; 2012.

Overweight: What Kids Say: What's Really Causing the Childhood Obesity Epidemic. 2nd ed. Robert A. Pretlow. eHealth International, Inc. Printed by CreateSpace, North Charleston, 2010. *www.weigh2rock.com*

Positive Parenting: Raising Healthy Children from Birth to Three Years. Alvin N. Eden. New York: Hatherleigh Press; 2007.

Reports

American Academy of Pediatrics, American Public Health Association, and National Resource Center for Health and Safety in Child Care and Early Education. 2012. *Preventing Childhood Obesity in Early Care and Education: Selected Standards from Caring for Our Children: National Health and Safety Performance Standards; Guidelines for Early Care and Education Programs*, 3rd ed. nrckids.org/CFOC3/PDFVersion/preventing_obesity.pdf

Institute of Medicine. *Early Childhood Obesity Prevention Policies*. Washington, DC: The National Academies Press; 2011.

Institute of Medicine. *Preventing Childhood Obesity: Health in the Balance*. Washington, DC: The National Academies Press; 2005.

National Association for Sport and Physical Education. *Active Start: A Statement of Physical Activity Guidelines for Children From Birth to Age 5*. 2nd ed. Reston, VA: National Association for Sport and Physical Education; 2009.

Websites

www.babybuilders.com: An exercise program for birth-to-walking infants that helps babies begin a lifestyle of fitness. Baby Builders is available in English, Spanish and French.

www.choosemyplate.gov: Learn how to build a meal by putting nutritious foods from all the food groups on your plate. For health and nutrition information about breastfeeding, visit:

www.choosemyplate.gov/pregnancy-breastfeeding.html

www.dontshake.org: The National Center on Shaken Baby Syndrome offers educational materials on coping with crying and the dangers of shaking a baby.

www.eatright.org: Website of the Academy of Nutrition and Dietetics that includes timely health and nutrition information for consumers and health professionals. It includes a national directory to help you find a registered dietitian nutritionist near you.

www.healthychildren.org: American Academy of Pediatrics website for parents that addresses children's health, fitness and nutrition. The section on babies from birth to 12 months includes information on breastfeeding, feeding and nutrition, and sleep.

justtherightbyte.com: Insightful blog by pediatric nutritionist and registered dietitian Jill Castle, who is also the co-author of *Fearless Feeding: How to Raise Healthy Eaters from High Chair to High School.*

www.kidsinthehouse.com: Website with thousands of short videos by experts on parenting. The Kids in the House collection includes infancy and offers 16 videos on childhood obesity featuring Dr. Barbara J. Moore, President and CEO of Shape Up America!®

www.raisehealthyeaters.com: Popular blog by family nutrition expert and registered dietitian Maryann Jacobsen, who is also the co-author of *Fearless Feeding: How to Raise Healthy Eaters from High Chair to High School.*

www.shapeup.org: Website of Shape Up America!®, a nonprofit organization that provides information on how to achieve and maintain a healthy weight for life.

Appendix C

References

Introduction

Cunningham SA, Kramer MR, Narayan KM. Incidence of childhood obesity in the United States. *New Engl J Med*. 2014;370(5):403-411.

Trust for America's Health and Robert Wood Johnson Foundation. *F as in Fat: How Obesity Threatens America's Future 2013*. Issue Report, August 2013.

Flores G, Lin H. Factors predicting overweight in US kindergartners. *Am J Clin Nutr*. 2013;97(6):1178-1187.

Birch LL, Anzman-Frasca S, Paul IM. Starting early: obesity prevention during infancy. In: Drewnowski A, Rolls BJ, eds. *Obesity Treatment and Prevention: New Directions*. Nestle Nutr Inst Workshop Ser. Nestec Ltd., Vevey/S. Karger AG., Basel, Switzerland; 2012;73:81-94.

Pretlow RA. *Overweight: What Kids Say: What's Really Causing the Childhood Obesity Epidemic*. 2nd ed. eHealth International, Inc. Printed by CreateSpace, North Charleston, 2010.

Taveras EM, Gillman MW, Kleinman KP, Rich-Edwards JW, Rifas-Shiman SL. Reducing racial/ethnic disparities in childhood obesity: the role of early life risk factors. *JAMA Pediatr*. 2013;167(8):731-738.

Chapter 1

American Academy of Pediatrics. AAP policy on breastfeeding and use of human milk. American Academy of Pediatrics website. *www2.aap.org/breastfeeding/policyOnBreastfeedingAndUseOfHumanMilk.html* Accessed January 13, 2014.

Centers for Disease Control and Prevention. Division of Nutrition, Physical Activity and Obesity, National Center for Chronic Disease Prevention and Health Promotion. Vitamin D supplementation. Centers for Disease Control and Prevention website. *www.cdc.gov/breastfeeding/recommendations/vitamin_d.htm* Updated October 20, 2009. Accessed January 13, 2014.

Belfort MB, Rifas-Shiman SL, Kleinman KP, et al. Infant feeding and childhood cognition at ages 3 and 7 years: Effects of breastfeeding duration and exclusivity. *JAMA Pediatr*. 2013;167(9):836-844.

Mortensen EL, Michaelsen KF, Sanders SA, Reinisch JM. The association between duration of breastfeeding and adult intelligence. *JAMA*. 2002;287(18):2365-2371.

Hussain SS, Bloom SR. The regulation of food intake by the gut-brain axis: implications for obesity. *Int J Obes*. 2013;37(5):625-633.

Vasselli JR. Appetite and body weight regulation. In: Akabas SR, Lederman SA, Moore BJ, eds. *Textbook of Obesity: Biological, Psychological and Cultural Influences*. West Sussex, UK: Wiley-Blackwell;2012:181-195.

Bouret SG. Developmental origins of obesity: energy balance pathways—appetite. The role of developmental plasticity of the hypothalamus. In: Gillman MW, Poston L, eds. *Maternal Obesity*. Cambridge, UK: Cambridge University Press;2012.

Plagemann A, Harder T, Brunn M, et al. Hypothalamic proopiomelanocortin promoter methylation becomes altered by early overfeeding: an epigenetic model of obesity and the metabolic syndrome. *J Physiol*. 2009;587(20):4963-4976.

Farooqi IS, Jebb SA, Langmack G, Lawrence E, Cheetham CH, Prentice AM, Hughes IA, McCamish MA, O'Rahilly S. Effects of recombinant leptin therapy in a child with congenital leptin deficiency. *N Engl J Med*. 1999;341(12):879-884.

Tellez LA, Medina S, Han W, et al. A gut lipid messenger links excess dietary fat to dopamine deficiency. *Science*. 2013;341(6147):800-802.

Casabiell X, Pineiro V, Tome MA, et al. Presence of leptin in colostrum and/or breast milk from lactating mothers: a potential role in the regulation of neonatal food intake. *J Clin Endocrinol Metab*. 1997;82(12):4270-4273.

Elmquist JK, Maratos-Flier E, Saper CB, Flier JS. Unraveling the central nervous system pathways underlying responses to leptin. *Nat Neurosci*. 1998;1(6):445-450.

Luo ZC, Nuyt AM, Delvin E, et al. Maternal and fetal leptin, adiponectin levels and association with fetal insulin sensitivity. *Obesity*. 2013;21(1):210-216.

Palou A, Pico C. Leptin intake during lactation prevents obesity and affects food intake and food preferences in later life. *Appetite*. 2009; 52(1):249-252.

Karatas Z, Durmus Aydogdu S, Dinleyici EC, Colak O, Dogruel N. Breastmilk ghrelin, leptin, and fat levels changing foremilk to hindmilk: is that important for self-control of feeding? *Eur J Pediatr*. 2011;170(10):1273-1280.

Dundar NO, Dundar B, Cesur G, Yilmaz N, Sutcu R, Ozguner F. Ghrelin and adiponectin levels in colostrum, cord blood and maternal serum. *Pediatr Int*. 2010;52(4):622-625.

Moller LM, de Hoog MLA, van Eijsden M, Gemke RJ, Vrijkotte TG. Infant nutrition in relation to eating behaviour and fruit and vegetable intake at age 5 years. *Brit. J Nutr*. 2013;109:564-571.

Mennella JA, Beauchamp GK. Flavor experiences during formula feeding are related to preferences during childhood. *Early Hum Dev*. 2002;68(2):71-82.

Institute of Medicine. *The Human Microbiome, Diet, and Health: Workshop Summary*. Washington, DC: The National Academies Press; 2013.

Ridaura VK, Faith JJ, Rey FE, et al. Gut microbiota from twins discordant for obesity modulate metabolism in mice. *Science*. 2013;341(6150):1241214.

Kalliomaki M, Collado MC, Salminen S, Isolauri E. Early differences in fecal microbiota composition in children may predict overweight. *Am J Clin Nutr*. 2008;87(3):534-538.

Chapter 2

American Academy of Pediatrics Policy Statement. Section on Breastfeeding. Breastfeeding and the use of human milk. Pediatrics. 2012; 129(3):e827-841. *pediatrics.aappublications.org/content/129/3/e827.full#content-block*

Centers for Disease Control and Prevention. Division of Nutrition and Physical Activity. Research to Practice Series No. 4: Does breastfeeding reduce the risk of pediatric overweight? Atlanta: Centers for Disease Control and Prevention; 2007. *www.cdc.gov/nccdphp/dnpa/nutrition/pdf/breastfeeding_r2p.pdf* Accessed January 26, 2013.

Centers for Disease Control and Prevention. Division of Nutrition, Physical Activity and Obesity, National Center for Chronic Disease Prevention and Health Promotion. Vitamin D supplementation. Centers for Disease Control and Prevention website. *www.cdc.gov/breastfeeding/recommendations/vitamin_d.htm* Updated October 20, 2009. Accessed January 13, 2014.

Grummer-Strawn LM, Mei Z; Centers for Disease Control and Prevention Pediatric Nutrition Surveillance System. Does breastfeeding protect against pediatric overweight? Analysis of longitudinal data from the Centers for Disease Control and Prevention Pediatric Nutrition Surveillance System. *Pediatrics.* 2004;113(2):e81-86.

Shape Up America!® website BMI calculator. *www.shapeup.org* Accessed January 26, 2014.

National Center for Chronic Disease Prevention and Health Promotion, Division of Nutrition, Physical Activity, and Obesity. CDC Vital Signs—Hospital support for breastfeeding. Centers for Disease Control and Prevention website. *www.cdc.gov/VitalSigns/Breastfeeding/index.html?s_cid=tw_ob497* Updated August 2, 2011. Accessed January 13, 2014.

Centers for Disease Control and Prevention. Vital signs: hospital practices to support breastfeeding—United States, 2007–2009. *MMWR.* 2011;60(30):1020-1025.

Brodribb W, Kruske S, Miller YD. Baby-friendly hospital accreditation, in-hospital care practices, and breastfeeding. *Pediatrics*. 2013;131(4):685-692.

Baby-friendly USA. Baby-friendly hospital initiative. Baby-friendly USA website. *https://www.babyfriendlyusa.org/about-us/baby-friendly-hospital-initiative* Accessed January 15, 2014.

Grummer-Strawn LM, Scanlon KS, Fein SB. Infant feeding and feeding transitions during the first year of life. *Pediatrics*. 2008;122(Supplement 2):S36-S42.

Trent. How much money does breastfeeding really save? The Simple Dollar website. *www.thesimpledollar.com/how-much-money-does-breastfeeding-really-save* Published March 4, 2007. Accessed January 15, 2014.

Li R, Fein SB, Grummer-Strawn LM. Do infants fed from bottles lack self-regulation of milk intake compared with directly breastfed infants? *Pediatrics*. 2010;125(6):e1386-e1393.

Dietz WH, Stern L, eds. *Nutrition: What Every Parent Needs to Know*. 2nd ed. Elk Grove Village, IL: American Academy of Pediatrics; 2012.

Lewis T, Amini F, Lannon R. *A General Theory of Love*. New York: First Vintage Edition; 2001.

Chapter 3

Birch LL, Anzman-Frasca S, Paul IM. Starting early: obesity prevention during infancy. In: Drewnowski A, Rolls BJ, eds. *Obesity Treatment and Prevention: New Directions*. Nestle Nutr Inst Workshop Ser. Nestec Ltd., Vevey/S. Karger AG., Basel, Switzerland; 2012;73:81-94.

Grummer-Strawn LM, Scanlon KS, Fein SB. Infant feeding and feeding transitions during the first year of life. *Pediatrics*. 2008;122(Supplement 2):S36-S42.

Institute of Medicine. *Early Childhood Obesity Prevention Policies*. Washington, DC: The National Academies Press; 2011.

Institute of Medicine. *Preventing Childhood Obesity: Health in the Balance.* Washington, DC: The National Academies Press; 2005.

Chapter 4

Clayton HB, Li R, Perrine CG, Scanlon KS. Prevalence and reasons for introducing infants early to solid foods: variations by milk feeding type. *Pediatrics.* 2013;131(4):e1108-1114.

Desai M, Beall M, Ross MG. Developmental origins of obesity: programmed adipogenesis. *Curr Diab Rep.* 2013;13(1):27-33.

Ferris AG, Vilhjalmsdottir LB, Beal VA, Pellett PL. Diets in the first six months of infants in western Massachusetts. II. Semi-solid foods. *J Am Diet Assoc.* 1978; 72(2):160-163.

United States Department of Agriculture, Food and Nutrition Service. Feeding solid foods, chapter 7. In: *Feeding Infants: A Guide for Use in the Child Nutrition Programs. www.fns.usda.gov/tn/feeding-infants-guide-use-child-nutrition-programs* Published July 1, 2002. Updated February 12, 2014. Accessed February 14, 2014.

United States Department of Agriculture. Feeding your baby in the first year. WIC Works website. *wicworks.nal.usda.gov/wicworks/Topics/infantfeedingtipsheet.pdf* Accessed February 14, 2014.

Flores G, Lin H. Factors predicting overweight in US kindergartners. *Am J Clin Nutr.* 2013;97:1178-1187.

Siega-Riz AM, Deming DM, Reidy KC, Fox MK, Condon E, Briefel RR. Food consumption patterns of infants and toddlers: where are we now? *J Am Diet Assoc.* 2010;110(12 Suppl):S38-S51.

Zhu H, Pollock NK, Kotak I, Gutin B, et al. Dietary sodium, adiposity and inflammation in healthy adolescents. *Pediatrics.* 2014 Mar;133(3):e635-642.

Rolland-Cachera MF, Maillot M, Deheeger M, Souberbielle JC, Peneau S, Hercberg S. Association of nutrition in early life with body fat and serum leptin at adult age. *Int J Obesity*. 2013;37(8):1116-1122.

Poti JM, Popkin BM. Trends in energy intake among US children by eating location and food source, 1977-2006. *J Am Diet Assoc*. 2011;111(8):1156-1164.

Chapter 5

Plagemann A, Harder T, Rodekamp E, Kohlhoff R. Rapid neonatal weight gain increases risk of childhood overweight in offspring of diabetic mothers. *J Perinat Med*. 2012;40(5):557-563.

Centers for Disease Control and Prevention, National Center for Health Statistics. WHO growth standards are recommended for use in the U.S. for infants and children 0–2 years of age. Data tables. *www.cdc.gov/growthcharts/who_charts.htm* Updated Sept 9, 2010. Accessed January 25, 2014.

Li R, Magadia J, Fein SB, Grummer-Strawn LM. Risk of bottle-feeding for rapid weight gain during the first year of life. *Arch Pediatr Adolesc Med*. 2012;166(5):431-436.

Li R, Fein SB, Grummer-Strawn LM. Association of breastfeeding intensity and bottle-emptying behaviors at early infancy with infants' risk for excess weight at late infancy. *Pediatrics*. 2008;122(Suppl 2):S77-S84.

Taveras EM, Rifas-Shiman SL, Belfort MB, Kleinman KP, Oken E, Gillman MW. Weight status in the first 6 months of life and obesity at 3 years of age. *Pediatrics*. 2009;123(4):1177-1183.

Tijhuis MJ, Doets EL, Vonk Noordegraaf-Schouten M. Extensive literature search and review as preparatory work for the evaluation of the essential composition of infant and follow-on formulae and growing-up milk. European Food Safety Authority supporting publication 2014:EN-551. *www.efsa.europa.eu/it/search/doc/551e.pdf* Accessed January 27, 2014.

Promoting Healthy Nutrition, Theme Five. In Hagan JF, Shaw JS, Duncan PM, eds. *Bright Futures: Guidelines for Health Supervision of Infants, Children, and Adolescents*, 3rd ed. Elk Grove Village, IL: American Academy of Pediatrics; 2008. *brightfutures.aap.org/3rd_edition_guidelines_and_pocket_guide.html* Accessed January 27, 2014.

Whitaker RC, Gooze RA. Nutrition and physical activity. In: Odom SL, Pungello EP, Gardner-Neblett N, eds. *Infants, Toddlers and Poverty: Research Implications for Early Child Care*. New York: Guilford Press;2012.

Flores G, Lin H. Factors predicting overweight in US kindergartners. *Am J Clin Nutr*. 2013;97:1178-1187.

Chapter 6

Dewar G. Infant sleep problems: a guide for the science-minded parent. Parenting Science website. *www.parentingscience.com/infant-sleep-problems.html* Updated March 2008. Accessed January 30, 2014.

Gortmaker SL, Must A, Sobol AM, Peterson K, Colditz GA, Dietz WH. Television viewing as a cause of increasing obesity among children in the United States, 1986-1990. *Arch Pediatr Adolesc Med*. 1996;150(4):356-362.

Andersen RE, Crespo CJ, Barlett SJ, Cheskin LC, Pratt M. Relationship of physical activity and television watching with body weight and level of fatness among children: results from the Third National Health and Nutrition Examination Survey. *JAMA*. 1998;279(12):938-942.

Robinson TN. Reducing children's television viewing to prevent obesity: a randomized controlled trial. *JAMA*. 1999;282(16):1561-1567.

Taveras EM, Gillman MW, Kleinman KP, Rich-Edwards JW, Rifas-Shiman SL. Reducing racial/ethnic disparities in childhood obesity: the role of early life risk factors. *JAMA Pediatr*. 2013;167(8):731-738.

Institute of Medicine. *Early Childhood Obesity Prevention Policies*. Washington, DC: The National Academies Press; 2011.

Birch LL, Anzman-Frasca S, Paul IM. Starting early: obesity prevention during infancy. In: Drewnowski A, Rolls BJ, eds. *Obesity Treatment and Prevention: New Directions*. Nestle Nutr Inst Workshop Ser. Nestec Ltd., Vevey/S. Karger AG., Basel, Switzerland; 2012;73:81-94.

Chapter 7

Whitaker RC, Gooze RA. Nutrition and physical activity. In: Odom SL, Pungello EP, Gardner-Neblett N, eds. *Infants, Toddlers and Poverty: Research Implications for Early Child Care*. New York: Guilford Press; 2012.

Flores G, Lin H. Factors predicting overweight in US kindergartners. *Am J Clin Nutr*. 2013;97:1178-1187.

Institute of Medicine. *Early Childhood Obesity Prevention Policies*, Washington, DC: The National Academies Press; 2011.

Eden AN. *Positive Parenting: Raising Healthy Children from Birth to Three Years*. New York: Hatherleigh Press; 2007.

Taveras EM, Gillman MW, Kleinman KP, Rich-Edwards JW, Rifas-Shiman SL. Reducing racial/ethnic disparities in childhood obesity: the role of early life risk factors. *JAMA Pediatr*. 2013;167(8):731-738.

Birch LL, Anzman-Frasca S, Paul IM. Starting early: obesity prevention during infancy. In: Drewnowski A, Rolls BJ, eds. *Obesity Treatment and Prevention: New Directions*. Nestle Nutr Inst Workshop Ser. Nestec Ltd., Vevey/S. Karger AG., Basel, Switzerland; 2012;73:81-94.

Chapter 8

Moore BJ, Greenwood MRC. Pregnancy and Weight Gain. In: Brownell KD, Fairburn CG, eds. *Eating Disorders and Obesity: A Comprehensive Handbook*. New York: Guilford Press; 1995:51-55.

Lederman SA. The relation of pregnancy and lactation to obesity development in the mother and child. In: Akabas SR, Lederman SA, Moore BJ, eds. *Textbook of Obesity: Biological, Psychological and Cultural Influences*. West Sussex, UK: Wiley-Blackwell; 2012:181-195.

Dewey KG, Heinig MJ, Nommsen LA. Maternal weight-loss patterns during prolonged lactation. *Am J Clin Nutr*. 1993;58(2):162-166.

Lederman SA. Influence of lactation on body weight regulation. *Nutr Rev*. 2004; 62(7 Pt 2): S112-119.

Chapter 9

Gaffney KF, Kitsantas P, Brito A, Swamidoss CS. Postpartum depression, infant feeding practices, and infant weight gain at six months of age. *J Pediatr Health Care*. 2014;28(1):43-50.

Murphy PK, Wagner CL. Vitamin D and mood disorders among women: an integrative review. *J Midwifery Womens Health*. 2008;53(5):440-446.

Odom ED, Li R, Scanlon KS, Perrine CG, Grummer-Strawn L. Reasons for earlier than desired cessation of breastfeeding. *Pediatrics*. 2013;131(3);e726-732.

Swinney B. *Eating Expectantly: Practical Advice for Healthy Eating Before, During and After Pregnancy*. 4th ed. El Paso, TX: Healthy Food Zone Media; 2013.

Devlieger RG, Guelinckx I. Pre-pregnancy bariatric surgery: improved fertility and pregnancy outcome? In: Gillman MW, Poston L, ed. *Maternal Obesity*. Cambridge, UK: Cambridge University Press; 2012: 209-221.

Harris AA, Barger MK. Specialized care for women pregnant after bariatric surgery. *J Midwifery Womens Health*. 2010;55(6):529–539.

Dao MC, Sen S, Iyer C, Klebenov D, Meydani SN. Obesity during pregnancy and fetal iron status: is hepcidin the link? *J Perinatol*. 2013;33:177-181.

Mennella, JA. Regulation of milk intake after exposure to alcohol in mothers' milk. *Alcohol Clin Exp Res.* 2001;25(4):590-593.

Mennella JA, Beauchamp GK. Beer, breast feeding and folklore. *Dev Psychobiol.* 1993;26(8):459-466.

National Institutes of Health, National Institute on Alcohol Abuse and Alcoholism. Mennella J. Alcohol's Effect on Lactation. National Institute on Alcohol Abuse and Alcoholism website. *pubs.niaaa.nih.gov/publications/arh25-3/230-234.htm* Accessed February 2, 2014.

Mennella JA, Garcia-Gomez PL. Sleep disturbances after acute exposure to alcohol in mothers' milk. *Alcohol.* 2001;25(3):153-158.

Mennella JA, Yourshaw LM, Morgan LK. Breastfeeding and smoking: short term effects on infant feeding and sleep. *Pediatrics.* 2007;120(3):497-502.

Centers for Disease Control and Prevention, Office on Smoking and Health, National Center for Chronic Disease Prevention and Health Promotion, Health Effects of Secondhand Smoke. Centers for Disease Control and Prevention website. *www.cdc.gov/tobacco/data_statistics/fact_sheets/secondhand_smoke/health_effects* Updated Jun 10, 2013. Accessed February 2, 2014.

Morandi A, Meyre D, Lobbens S, et al. Estimation of newborn risk for child or adolescent obesity: lessons from longitudinal birth cohorts. *PLOS One.* 2012; 7(11):e49919.

Davis MM, McGonagle K, Schoeni RF, Stafford F. Grandparental and parental obesity influences on childhood overweight: implications for primary care practice. *J Am Board Fam Med.* 2008;21(6):549-554.

Whitaker KL, Jarvis MJ, Beeken RJ, Boniface D, Wardle J: Comparing maternal and paternal intergenerational transmission of obesity risk in a large population-based sample. *Am J Clin Nutr.* 2010;91:1560–1567.

Dietz WH, Stern L, eds. *Nutrition: What Every Parent Needs to Know.* 2nd ed. Elk Grove Village, IL: American Academy of Pediatrics; 2012.

Chapter 10

Birch LL, Anzman-Frasca S, Paul IM. Starting early: obesity prevention during infancy. In: Drewnowski A, Rolls BJ, eds. *Obesity Treatment and Prevention: New Directions*. Nestle Nutr Inst Workshop Ser. Nestec Ltd., Vevey/S. Karger AG., Basel, Switzerland; 2012;73:81-94.

Moore BJ, Frame IJ, Baehr N. Preventing childhood obesity: it takes a nation. In: Akabas SR, Lederman SA, Moore BJ, eds. *Textbook of Obesity: Biological, Psychological and Cultural Influences*. West Sussex, UK: Wiley-Blackwell; 2012:424-462.

Colophon

The paperback edition of *Fit from the Start* was designed and typeset by *IndieBookLauncher.com*.

The body text is set in Minion 12pt. The chapter headings are set in Verb. URLs and table headings are set in Myriad.

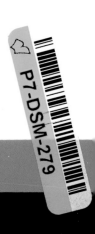